Tai Chi

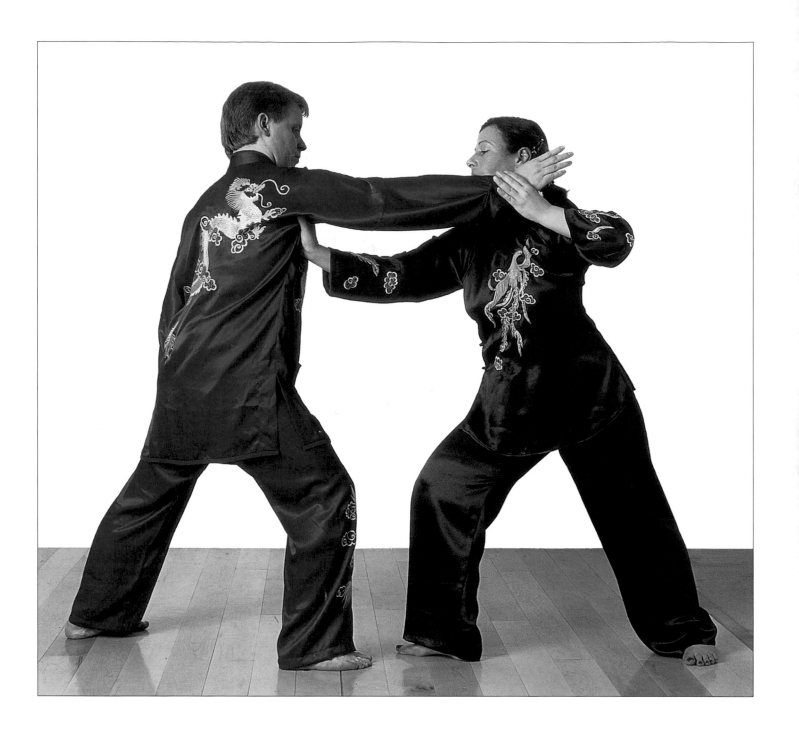

Tai Chi

A practical introduction

RAYMOND PAWLETT

Oceana

An Oceana Book

This book is designed and produced by
Oceana Books
The Old Brewery
6 Blundell Street
London N7 9BH

ISBN 1-86160-280-4

QUMAIT

Project Manager: Rebecca Kingsley / Joyce Bentley
Project Editor: Maria Costantino
Photographer: Paul Forrester
Editor: Sarah Harris
Designer: Ned Hoste

Manufactured in Singapore by Pica Graphics
Printed in Singapore by Star Standard Industries Pte. Ltd.

This book is not intended as a substitute for the advice of a health care
professional. If you have any reason to believe you have a condition
which affects your health, you must seek professional advice. Consult a
qualified health care professional, aromatherapist or your doctor before
starting.

c o n t e n t s

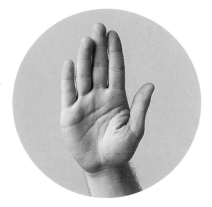

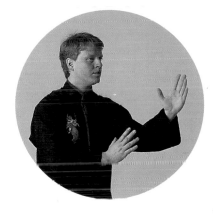

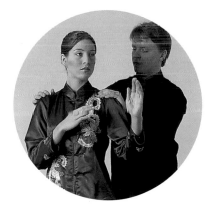

introduction to
Tai Chi

WHAT IS TAI CHI CHUAN

What is Tai Chi Chuan? As you learn more about Tai Chi, your definition will change. Your perceptions will lean more towards one aspect of the art at different times.

As an exercise, put down this book now and on a blank piece of paper define in your own terms what YOU perceive Tai Chi Chuan to be. The references can be as direct or as abstract as you like, as long as it means something to YOU. This is a useful exercise that should be done several times during your Tai Chi development.

It is true that trying to define Tai Chi Chuan can never be totally accurate — as the Taoists have said for many years, the essence of a thing is unnameable, and it is easier to describe what a thing is not rather than what it is. It is however a useful exercise and reference point.

Fundamentally Tai Chi Chuan stems from three cores of Chinese knowledge which are:

(1) Martial arts
(2) Healing arts
(3) Philosophy

As a martial art, Tai Chi Chuan employs softness rather than strength. This can be likened to the flexible strength of a willow tree in a storm, compared to the rigidity of a great oak tree that can be uprooted and blown over.

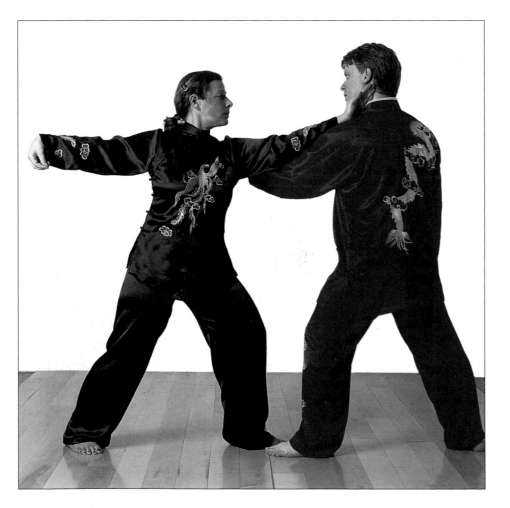

Tai Chi uses softness, rather than force, in its martial applications.

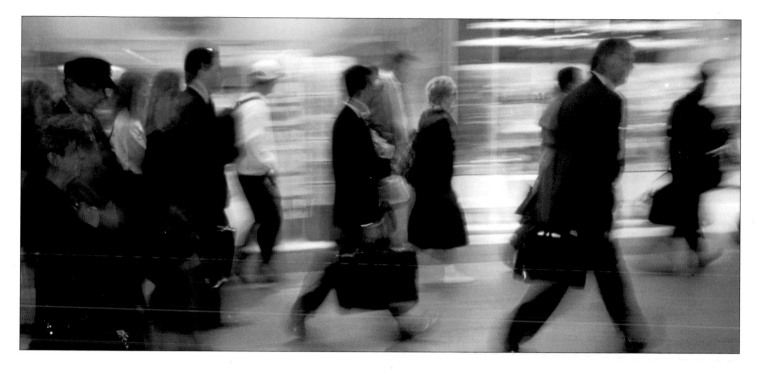

An example of this is yielding to re-direct a force rather than meeting it head-on. The re-direction will require very little physical effort whereas the head-on approach would need a greater force to neutralise the oncoming. Therefore using softness means that the strongest force will not necessarily win every time.

This is the meaning of the classic Tai Chi Chuan phrase, "use an ounce to stop a thousand pounds".

When you have started to experience and understand the martial arts aspect of Tai Chi Chuan, your energy level will reach a point at which it can be used for healing. The student will be able to sense and use energy for any of the various healing arts.

Behind the overall frame of Tai Chi Chuan, lies an understanding of the Universal forces of Yin and Yang. Whilst many people have seen the black and white Yin/Yang symbol, fewer are aware that it is actually called the Tai Chi symbol. By practising Tai Chi Chuan, you can learn about Yin and Yang through direct experience, rather than a theoretical knowledge gained from a book.

There is another quality of Tai Chi Chuan that should never leave us — it is fun. There should always be this kind of a soft enjoyment to your Tai Chi Chuan practice, which, when observed, will not look intimidating to children.

Tai Chi has many different angles of exploration. There are various styles of Tai Chi, and even different ways of doing the same style. Within any one style there will usually be elements of form (pattern) training, energy building exercises, healing, martial applications, pushing hands and weapons training to name but a few facets of the art.

In today's busy, stressful environment, Tai Chi can reduce tension and aid relaxation

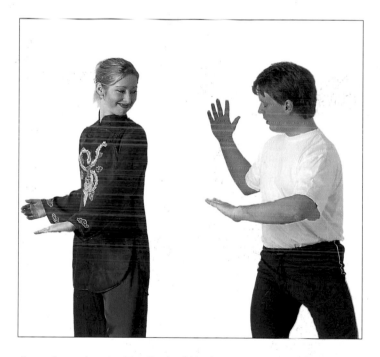

Remember — learning Tai Chi should be fun!

The style of Tai Chi explained in this book is the Yang style. In traditional Yang style Tai Chi, as practised by the Yang family, there are 103 moves in the form. This makes learning the whole of the form a somewhat daunting task for the beginner. It is for that reason that the Simplified, or Basic, Form was invented. It has only 24 movements, yet contains all of the essences of Tai Chi. It is the Simplified Form that is shown in this book. An advantage of learning the Yang style of Tai Chi is that it is the most common style in the world. Most cities or large towns will have a Tai Chi club somewhere, allowing you to train with more experienced Tai Chi people.

Intrinsic to Tai Chi is the idea of Energy. When we talk about energy in this context, we are talking about the internal Energy within the body — the Energy that stops us from simply being a collection of chemical reactions and gives us life itself. The Chinese name for this Energy is 'Chi'. The basic idea of Chi will be discussed in a later chapter.

The ancient Chinese Yin/Yang symbol has become a fashionable piece of graphic artwork in recent years. Most people will be familiar with the circular shape that is black on one side and white on the other. From the many who have seen the symbol or even have it on their T-shirts, relatively few will be aware that the symbol is called the Tai Chi symbol or the symbol of the 'Supreme Ultimate'.

What the symbol illustrates is the interaction between the universal forces of Yin and Yang. This is the foundation upon which the concepts and philosophy are based. The idea of Yin and Yang will also be expanded upon later.

The only real 'secret' to Tai Chi is that 'practice makes perfect'. The trouble with this is that with the best will in the world, it can be difficult to fit much Tai Chi into your day if you have other commitments. For this reason some tips towards getting the most out of your valuable practise time will be given at the end of the book.

Black and White are classic Tai Chi colours, representing the Yin and Yang symbol.

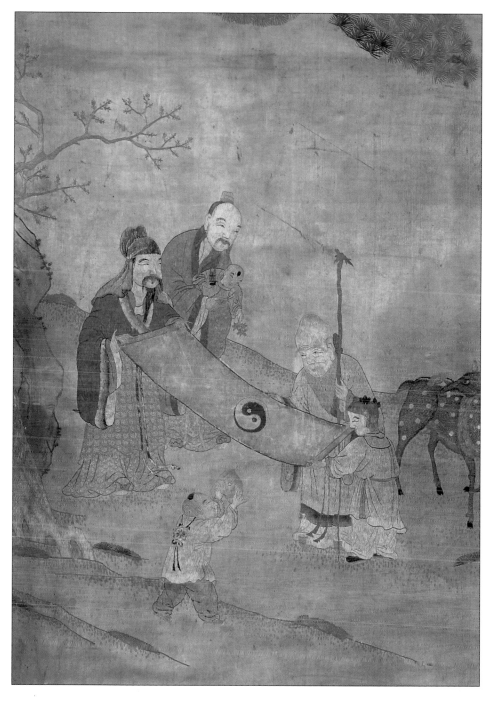

Tai Chi has its origins in ancient Chinese history and legend.

TAI CHI LEGENDS

The origins of Tai Chi Chuan have become clouded in the mists of time. There are various explanations as to where it originated, many of them involving ancient Chinese Alchemists or Taoists.

The history of Tai Chi is a valuable aid to learning the art because it can help to give a greater depth of understanding to the art. As with any practice that can trace its history back through the centuries, there are many myths and legends surrounding Tai Chi.

One of the most interesting stories claims that Tai Chi was presented to a Taoist monk in the form of a dream by 'extraterrestrials', with instructions for the form to be transmitted to humankind. Many of the stories cite the Wudang Mountain in China as being the place of origin for Tai Chi Chuan. The art is indeed still practised there in modern times.

Many of the old Chinese texts take the Taoist priest Zhang Sangfeng, who lived in the fifteenth century, as the originator of Tai Chi Chuan. He is said to have witnessed a struggle between a snake and a bird, which gave him the inspiration for Tai Chi Chuan. The bird was trying to eat the snake, but could not pick it up to do so. The reason for this was that the snake stayed soft and supple whilst the bird was trying to devour it. The snake managed to wriggle out of the bird's clutches and was able to live another day.

Some of the stories about the origins of Tai Chi Chuan may owe as much to human imagination as to fact. Like all of the Taoist stories, there is a grain of knowledge hidden within them.

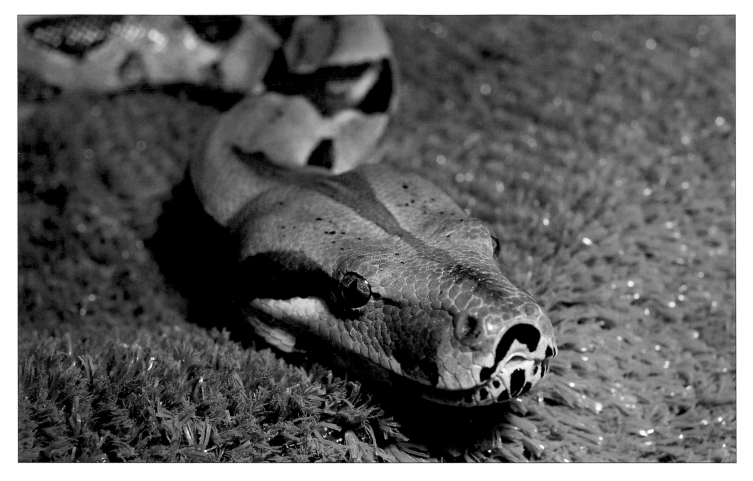

One of the earliest Tai Chi legends describes how the suppleness of the snake (softness) overcame the rigidity of the bird (strength).

The idea of receiving transmissions about Tai Chi Chuan in a dream can be interpreted as using meditation to reach different levels of consciousness. Meditation can teach valuable lessons about oneself and Tai Chi Chuan. The story is therefore highlighting the spiritual and meditative aspects of Tai Chi Chuan.

It may be that the legendary confrontation between the snake and the bird had very little to do with the actual origins of Tai Chi. In real life, some birds do manage to eat snakes without actually starving to death trying to catch them!

The real point of the legend is to present the idea that softness is able to overcome rigidity. Although the snake may have had a few knocks and bruises from the escapade, it eventually escaped. The lithe movements of the snake enabled it to avoid the stabbing and grabbing of the bird's beak and claws.

This would be analogous to a person who, when threatened by a stronger force, does not respond with another show of force, but remains soft and relaxed and yields to the attack. The opponent will therefore have very little to attack and will hopefully soon quit.

Yin and Yang

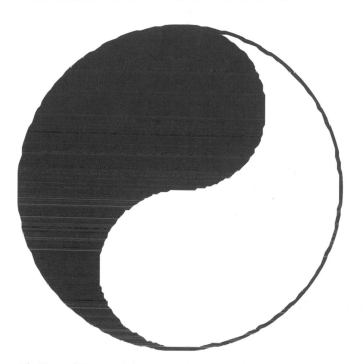

The Yin and Yang symbol represents the two complementary forces that make up our universe.

In Taoist cosmology, at the origin of the Universe there was an empty state called Wu Chi. Wu Chi simply means nothingness and is symbolised by an empty circle. In the original void, forces started to attract and repel each other. Eventually there were two different forces within the void. These two forces are known as Yin and Yang.

The Yin and Yang forces coalesced together with such density that matter formed. It is from this concentration of Yin and Yang forces into matter that the 'Ten Thousand Things' of the physical Universe were born. The phrase 'Ten Thousand Things' is not a literal phrase but is simply a large number used to represent all the individual items in the Universe.

The implication of this is that everything around us consists of Yin and Yang forces and contained within that are the origins of the universe. This worldview is not entirely at odds with the findings of modern physics. The theory that energy and matter are the same is also stated in Einstein's famous equation: $E = MC^2$

(Where E = energy, M = mass (or matter) and C = speed of light).

The idea of Yin and Yang forms the philosophical framework upon which Tai Chi was founded. The starting posture of the Tai Chi form is called the Wu Chi posture and symbolises nothingness, or emptiness. As the arms begin to lift, the internal forces of Yin and Yang are starting to define themselves. When the form starts to move, we are constantly using contraction and expansion (Yin and Yang). The movement of the form through the Yin and Yang energies is a microcosm of the Ten Thousand Things. At the end of the form, all energy returns to where it started from — the Wu Chi posture.

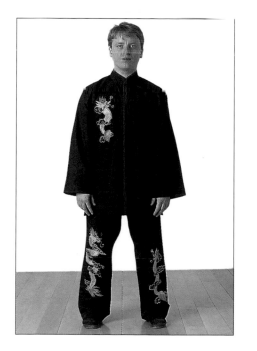

The Wu Chi posture both begins and ends the Tai Chi form.

Energy – Chi

The concept of Chi (or Qi) is central to Tai Chi and other healing and martial arts throughout the world. Chi has been the source of debate for centuries and will most probably stay that way for centuries yet to come.

One of the major causes for debate is that Chi is the non-physical, or etheric, part of a person. Some very learned individuals therefore dismiss the concept, as the etheric body is invisible to the untrained eye so they think that it cannot exist.

The fundamental view of the human body outlined by Chinese medicine states that the organisation of the energetic part of the human body precedes the organisation of the physical part of the human body. This means that movement of Chi brings about all thoughts, emotions and movements of the human body.

Another implication is that if a person can alter their own or somebody else's energetic body, then the state of mind or body can also be altered. Healers and martial artists who use Chi as a part of their processes will therefore be doing exactly that.

One of the aims of Tai Chi practise is to refine our Chi, and by refining the energetic body, refinements will also be made to our body, mind and spirit. In this way we will be healing ourselves.

There are different manifestations of Chi. An inanimate object has Chi, but has no life. This would mean that it has no 'Jing'. Jing is the manifestation of Chi that allows life to be present within a thing. A good example would be that a building would have its own Chi but no Jing.

A living thing has Jing. If a living thing has another quality of Chi called 'Shen', then it will have the capability of self-reflection. Traditional Chinese medicine believes that the only creatures capable of Shen are humans. People with a great amount of Shen will be capable of great self-reflection. Buddha would therefore have possessed large amounts of Shen.

Chi comes to us from three places. These are the Chi that we are born with, the Chi that we get from our food and the Chi that we get through breathing. If we stop getting enough of either food Chi or air Chi (we cannot alter birth Chi), we become ill. When practising Tai Chi, the breathing comes from the stomach. The reason for this is that our reservoir of Chi is situated in the stomach. When we breathe Chi into the stomach we top up our Chi and increase our vital Energy.

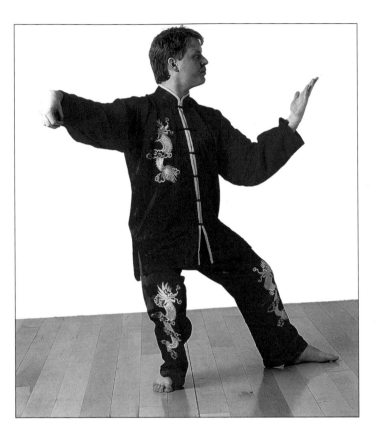

Through Tai Chi we can learn to control and enhance our Chi, or Energy.

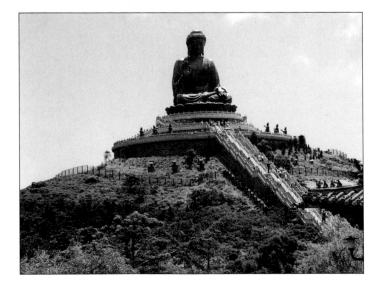

The meditative strength and serenity of Buddha represents great Shen.

Essences

The Ten Essences of Tai Chi are:

(1) Lift the head to raise the spirit
(2) Lower the shoulders to sink the elbows
(3) Curve the back and soften the chest
(4) Loosen the waist
(5) Be aware of weight distribution
(6) Co-ordinate the top half of the body with the bottom half of the body
(7) Continuity in movement
(8) Unite the mind (intent) with the body (frame)
(9) Use mind and not force
(10) Seek stillness within motion and motion within stillness

The Ten Essences were developed by Yang Cheng Fu to help his students understand the movements of the form. Yang Cheng Fu lived in China between 1883 and 1936. He adapted the Yang-style Tai Chi form to the series of movements we know today.

Since then the Ten Essences have become an invaluable learning aid to many exponents of the art. When fully understood, the Ten Essences define a type of body structure rather than trying to dictate actual moves. The Ten Essences can therefore be valuable knowledge to any Martial arts students (no matter what style), and even to dance students. When watching a well-trained dancer, one will usually be able to see the Essences in place.

The Essences can therefore be regarded as the building blocks of Tai Chi Chuan. If one of the Essences is not in place, the student will have great difficulty trying to reach any high skill level.

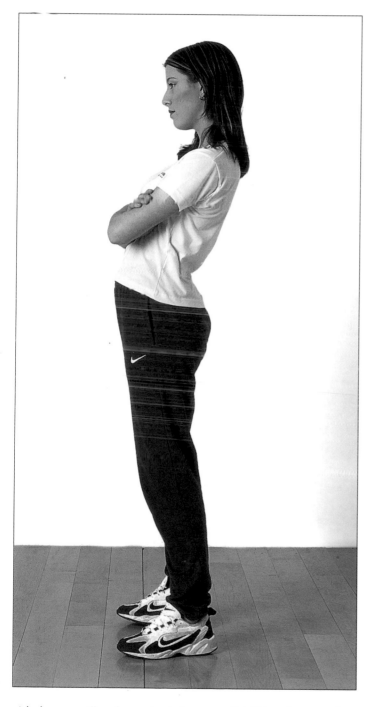

A bad posture will need correcting before correct Tai Chi can be practiced.

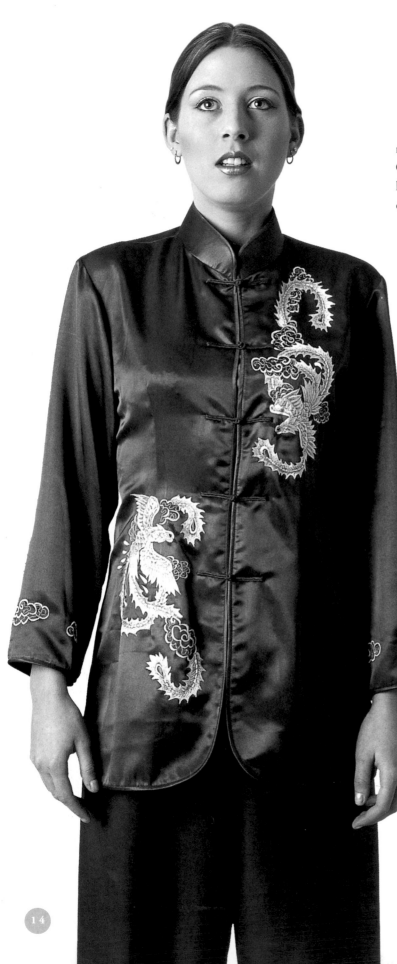

When Yang Cheng Fu developed the Essences, they were in no particular order. More recently Christopher Pei, a modern Tai Chi master of great reputation, has revisited the Ten Essences. He has shown that they can be rearranged into a chronological order of skill level. This means that it is helpful to work on the Essences in the order in which they come. A student's time is therefore better spent practising the first Essences in the form and gradually moving on to the latter ones, than working on the later Essences first. It follows then that one may be able to assess a Tai Chi practitioner's skill level in the art by observing which of the Essences are in place.

The first five Essences are physical Essences, which set up the conditions in the body for correct practise of Tai Chi Chuan. Without the physical conditions that are fulfilled by the first five Essences, one cannot successfully develop the last five Essences.

This would be similar to an architect trying to build a great building but having weak foundations. Sooner or later the building will topple, and will have to be re-built. It would have been better in the long run to have spent more time on the foundations. The architect could have then built higher without finishing with a pile of rubble. If the architect still wants to create his masterpiece, he will do no better unless he alters the foundations, so effectively he will have to start again. To avoid having to start again with Tai Chi, get the Essences correct in the first place and you will be able to build as high as you want.

The first of the five physical Essences starts at the head. The fifth finishes at the feet. It is therefore possible, once these essences have been understood, to use the Essences as a physical checklist at any point in the form to check posture.

Once the physical requirements of the first five Essences are in place, work will automatically begin on Essences six to ten. The key word to these essences is co-ordination. When we study Tai Chi Chuan, one of our

The Ten Essences can help correct a too-tense body.

aims can be co-ordination or strengthening the links between Mind, Body and Spirit.

This is indeed a lofty sounding goal, and needs explanation to become a practical piece of knowledge rather than yet more esoteric rhetoric.

When we are working on Essences six and seven, we are mostly working with the co-ordination of the upper and lower body. On eight and nine, we are uniting mind and body. On the last Essence, number ten, we are working mostly with Spirit.

The Ten Essences effectively form a 'map' which will help you to chart the previously unknown country of Body, Mind and Sprit. By working patiently and methodically, you will gain an understanding of the last Essences.

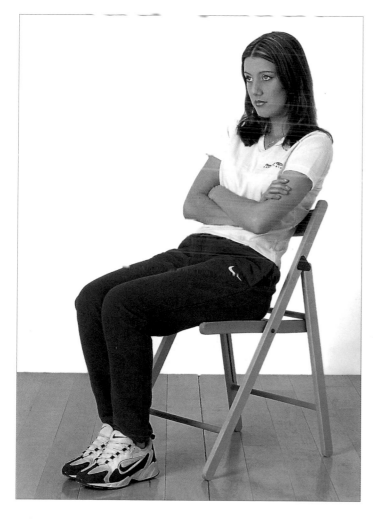

A bad posture can reflect a bad attitude.

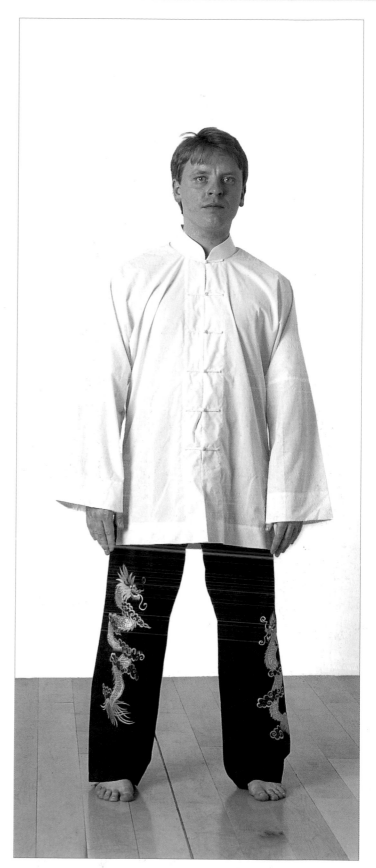

The Ten Essences co-ordinate the body's positioning and energies.

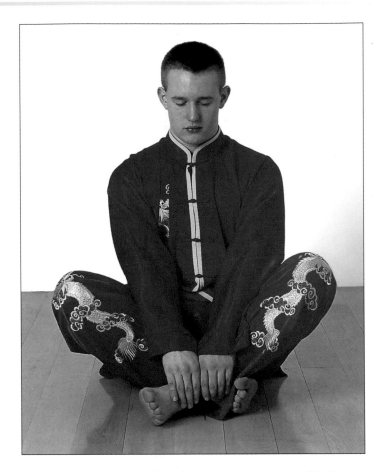

Achieving harmony between the body and mind is at the heart of the Ten Essences.

This then begs the question of what happens after the Tenth Essence. Will you know everything about Tai Chi? The answer to this question can actually be found in the first Essence, which refers to Spirit.

Originally you will have simply lifted the head. At first it will be difficult enough just to maintain this throughout the form. After working through the Essences, you will have made changes to your body, energy and understanding of the basics. You should now understand 'Lift the Head to Raise the Spirit' in a completely different way from when you started. The task now is to apply that new understanding to the Tai Chi form.

This is how the Ten Essences can be used as a tool for the continuous development of your Tai Chi Chuan.

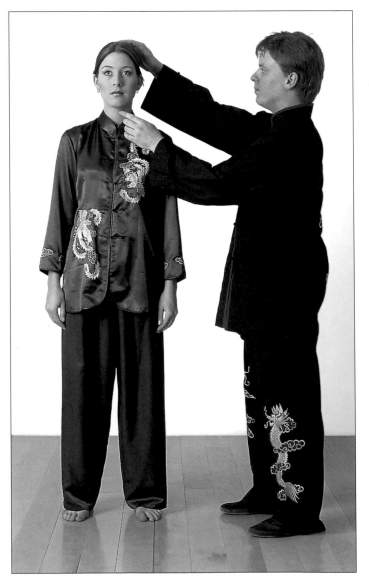

It may take time to achieve the correct stance, but it is worth persevering.

Ten Essences

(1) Lift the Head to Raise the Spirit

Next time that you are in a waiting room or other busy place, take a look at the people around you. You will probably see that many people are wandering around with their heads bowed, looking at either the floor or their shoes. The reasons for this can be varied; they could be ill, tired or sad.

To practise the first Essence, stand straight and hold the neck and head upright and relaxed. Imagine the mind concentrated together at the top of the head. This should be relaxed, otherwise the flow of Chi will be affected.

If your head is bowed, then your spirit cannot be high. Simply by straightening your back and lifting your head, the spirit will lift. A person who feels that they have 'the weight of the world on their shoulders' will not have good spirit. Next time you are feeling a bit like this, consider how you are holding your body and straighten up a bit to lift the spirit. In this way you are teaching yourself to 'walk tall'.

From a martial artist's point of view, this is probably the most important Essence. The first thing that two competitors will do is to look at each other. Imagine that one competitor has his head raised and is looking relaxed. Then imagine that the opponent only half looks up, and half looks downwards. The body language has already told you where to place your bets.

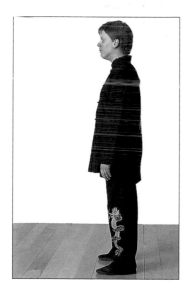

Stand straight and hold your head and neck upright, but relaxed.

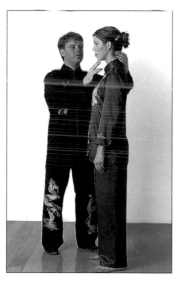

Lifting your head will lift your spirits.

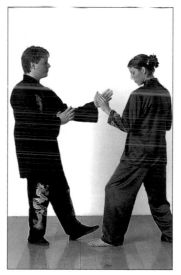

With the head bowed, an opponent looks defeated from the beginning.

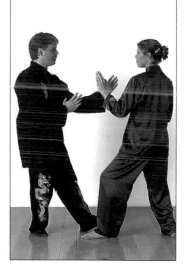

Now with the head raised, both opponents are evenly matched.

(2) LOWER THE SHOULDERS TO SINK THE ELBOWS

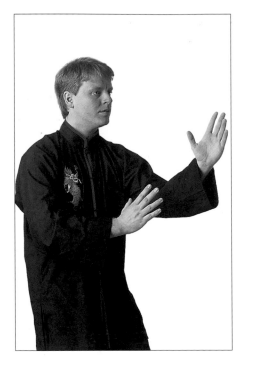

Here the shoulders are lowered, and the elbows dipped.

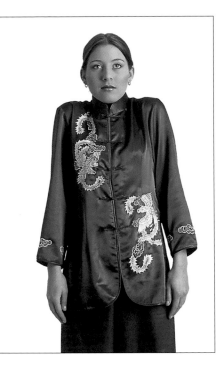

Holding your shoulders high for any length of time is a great strain.

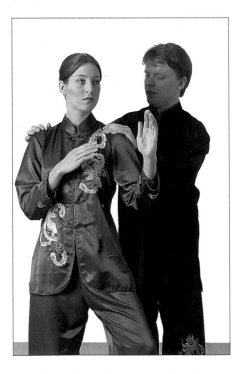

It will take effort to keep the shoulders relaxed.

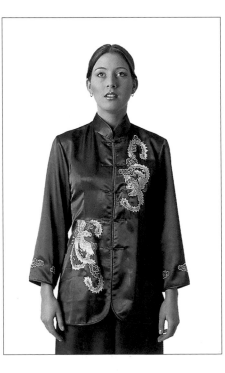

Once you can keep your shoulders lowered, you have enhanced your Energy.

In Tai Chi, there will always be a pairing of Yin and Yang. It follows that if the head is raised, then something must be lowered. If the shoulders are not lowered, energy will be trapped high up on the body and becomes useless.

Prove this to yourself by standing up and lifting the shoulders as high as you can for a couple of minutes. Try and lift your shoulders so high that they are touching your ears.

Then suddenly release them, and feel the relief. After a while it becomes a real physical strain to keep your shoulders high. On a smaller scale, even if your shoulders are only slightly raised, precious energy is simply being wasted.

For the martial artist, the basic mechanics illustrate the point. If the shoulders are high, the centre of gravity will be raised. For maximum stability in any structure, the centre of gravity should be low. It therefore makes sense that the person with the lower centre of gravity has a lower possibility of being knocked over.

A good tip for this is to try and keep the elbows pointing down to the floor. If the elbows are pointing down, then the shoulders will be down.

(3) SOFTEN THE CHEST – CURVE THE BACK

Stand to attention! Chin up! Shoulders back! Feet together!

This has become a part of the physical conditioning of our culture. Whether in the services, at school or simply picking the ideas up from the television, many people have similar body dynamics to this.

The opposite end of this scale is a slumped posture that pushes the abdomen forward, which affects the working of the internal organs.

These postures are not natural to us. They are learned by the body from such things as repetitive activities, imitation, emotional stress and physiological compensation for old injuries. Tai Chi teaches us to reprogram ourselves to be able to stand in a way that will not put any unwanted stresses and strains on the skeleton or the internal organs.

Instead of pulling the shoulders back, fold them forwards gently. Make sure that your back is straight, your head up and your shoulders down (from Essences one and two). Repeat the mental checks that you did whilst standing in the 'Attention!' posture.

You may now find that your breathing can become softer and that your abdomen will start to move with your breathing. The reason for this is that the Energy meridian for the lungs has become softer, thus allowing your breathing to become deeper. The important part of this meridian is at its end. This point lies just below your shoulders and needs to be relaxed to allow your breathing to relax.

When your breathing becomes relaxed, your body can become relaxed. Your skeleton itself will have less pressure on it from bad body posture, and your internal organs will also become less restricted.

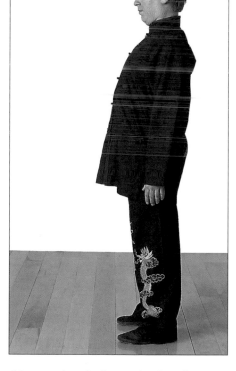

Many people make the mistake of standing to attention, puffing their chests out.

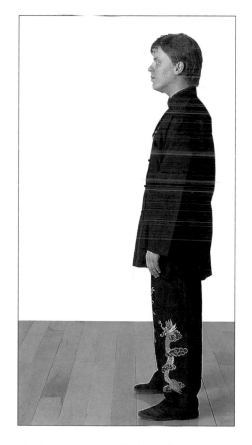

A relaxed posture with back straight is correct.

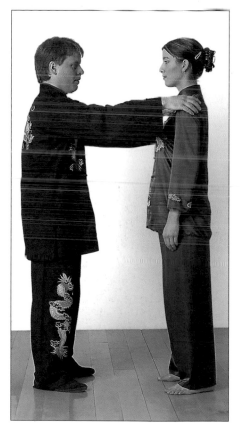

You may need help to achieve this posture.

(4) LOOSEN THE WAIST

When the physical requirements of the first three Essences have been attained, your body will have started to relax and become softer. This allows your breathing to sink to the Tan Tien.

The Tan Tien is a very important point within the Tai Chi system, as it is with other martial and healing arts. It is an invisible energy centre that is positioned just below the navel. Other names for is are the 'sea of Ki' or centre of the 'Hara'. These are both Japanese phrases for the same thing.

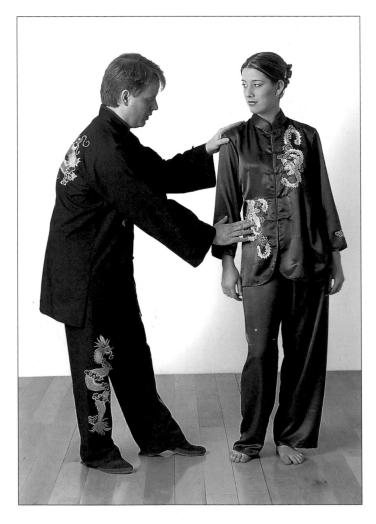

Loosening the waist completes the correct posture procedure for the upper body.

The important point is that the Tan Tien radiates energy out to the rest of the body. It can be felt and its effects observed, but it is not a physical entity that can be seen with normal vision.

Most people when they first see Tai Chi being performed notice the movement of the arms and legs. Indeed many Tai Chi practitioners only move the limbs. For Tai Chi to be done properly, the movement should come from the Tan Tien. Movement of the arms and legs within Tai Chi should be like ripples coming from the Tan Tien.

A useful piece of advice here is that when learning a new move in the Tai Chi (or re-learning an old one), do not be confused by the hands and feet. Try and see the body as a unified entity, with the centre of movement being the waist. Try and work out how to move the waist so that the desired movement happens. When Tai Chi moves are incorrectly executed, it is usually the waist that is wrong. You will save a great deal of time if you address your movement from the waist as soon as possible, rather than trying to work out where your hands and feet should be. The movement will then be more grounded and intuitive.

If your breathing sinks into the Tan Tien by using the first three Essences, then the Tan Tien will become stronger. This will allow the movements to be issued from your waist, or the Tan Tien. For this to happen, your waist must be free to move. If your waist will not allow this freedom of movement, the ripples on our pond of Energy will be more like throwing a pebble into mud. No energy will be allowed to travel outwards.

The first Essences effectively set up the conditions for the upper body. You have now moved down to the waist and are setting up conditions for the lower body. One thing that should have remained with you throughout is the idea of letting go of tension. Starting with the upper body, this release of tension continues at the waist. Some useful advice here is to let these processes happen gradually. Stiffness can be caused by many physical and physiological factors that will not disappear overnight. Only through diligent practice and patience will the rewards come.

This applies equally to the old habits that we are trying to undo and the new 'programming' that we are trying to download, using Tai Chi as the medium.

(5) BE AWARE OF WEIGHT DISTRIBUTION

To gain a feeling of what the Fifth Essence is teaching, stand for a while in a natural posture. At this moment you are not particularly concerned about what the stance is. You are simply looking at the feelings within the stance.

Give yourself a couple of minutes to settle down into the stance, and then start to go through the Essences that you have learnt so far. Lift up the crown of your head, but allow your chin to relax. Keep your back straight. Let your shoulders drop down, as if your hands are heavy. Fold your shoulders slightly forward and allow your breathing to soften. Relax your waist. Keep your spine straight and do not allow your bottom to poke out. Let your breathing become soft, so that when you breathe in, your abdomen comes out and when you breathe out, your abdomen comes in.

The top of your body and your trunk should now be fairly well lined up and relaxed. Now you need to check your knees and ankles. They should be relaxed. Never allow your knee joints to lock up. Make sure that the joints are relaxed by bending them slightly. Do not forget that your back has to be straight, even if your knees are bent, so do not tip your body forwards or backwards.

Now feel the weight in your feet. If you are in a balanced posture, your weight distribution should be divided equally between each foot. If this is not the case, try and correct your posture. You are now working with the Fifth Essence, which is the awareness of weight distribution.

Try playing with your weight distribution. Push the heel of your left foot into the floor gradually, so that the distribution changes from fifty-fifty to sixty-forty, then from sixty-forty to seventy-thirty and so on until all your weight is on your left leg. Try doing this exercise several times until you can change the weight distribution from foot to foot without altering the alignment of your body.

You may find that this exercise requires more effort than you anticipated. The reason for this is that altering the weight in the legs as you have just done is automatically altering the feeling of 'rooting'.

One of the reasons that Tai Chi is so popular is that it can reduce stress. Generally we have countless mental dialogues going through our minds, and we often do one thing while thinking about something else. The control taught by the proper practise of Tai Chi can slow down this sort of mental dialogue, enabling us be more focussed.

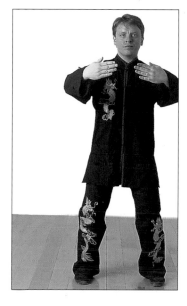

To achieve a balance, you must be aware of the weight in your feet.

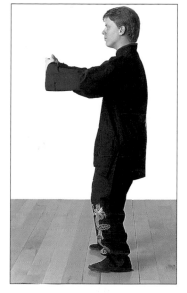

Practicing adjusting your weight distribution is vital for correct Tai Chi movements.

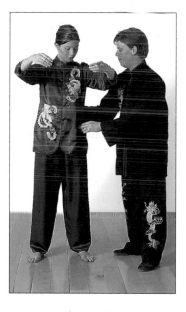

Getting the balance right can take time and effort.

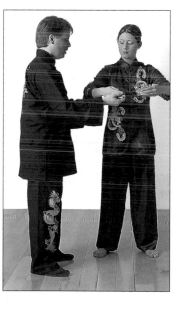

You may well need an instructor's help before mastering this technique.

(6) CO-ORDINATE THE TOP HALF OF THE BODY WITH THE BOTTOM

Imagine an army going into battle. This army has a problem at the moment. The trouble is that half the soldiers are at home watching the television. The remaining soldiers on the front line will not be as effective, because they have not managed to mobilise all their forces.

Mobilisation of the whole of the forces within the body is one of the fundamental requirements of Tai Chi. For example, during a push, the beginner will usually perform the push with the top half of the body only. This will mean that the bottom half of the body (where the strongest muscles are) is not used in the push.

The more experienced Tai Chi student, who can use the legs for the push, as well as the arms, will have a stronger technique. The reason for this is that the second student has managed to use the whole of the body, rather than just the top. This is why you must pay attention to the co-ordination of the upper and lower halves of your body.

This is quite easy to observe. When a move is coming forward, your knee should stop moving at the same time as your elbow. If one part of your body finishes before the other part, the co-ordination of your upper and lower body is at fault.

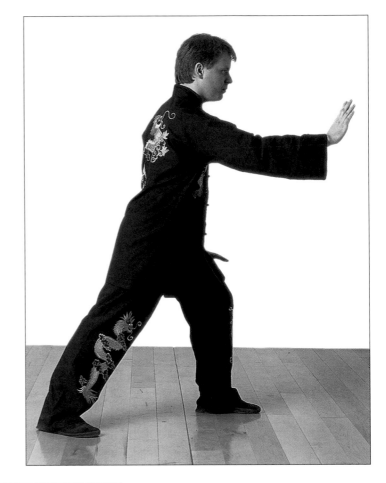

It is important to co-ordinate the different parts of the body. Here the legs and arms are balanced.

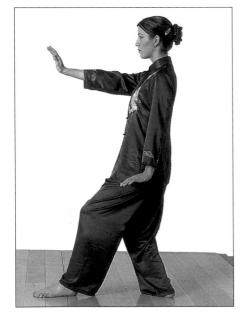

Here the balance is incorrect, as the back leg is bent.

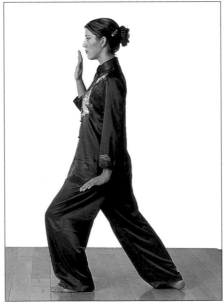

Again this shows incorrect balance, as the arms have not gone forward to balance the legs.

(7) CONTINUITY IN MOVEMENT

Think back to the army that we spoke of during the last Essence. This time they are more focussed. They are marching in the morning this time, so there is nothing to distract them from their task. Unfortunately, some of the soldiers stayed up rather late and are suffering from tiredness.

This tiredness gradually becomes all they can think about, so some of the soldiers stop for a short break, promising that they will catch up soon. This would obviously be a hazardous situation. There is nothing to gain from mobilising the whole army if they are not co-ordinated. The group of soldiers needs to be constantly in motion to be effective, otherwise there will still only be half of the army meeting any attack.

This same logic applies to Tai Chi. Once the body starts to move, it should stay moving. Different parts of the body will move at different speeds, but at no time should any part of the body stop so that another part can catch up.

This also shows how closely Essences six and seven are linked. If the movement is being generated from the waist, and the top and bottom halves of the body are co-ordinated, the movement will be continuous. If the legs are moving before the arms, or vice versa, one part of the body will have to stop so that the other can catch up, and the movement will not be continuous.

Co-ordinated movement allows the form to become soft and continuous and sets up the pre-requisites for Energy flow.

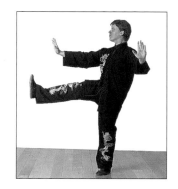

Achieving continuity means that the various parts of the body move in harmony.

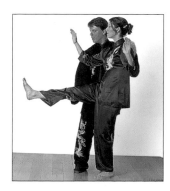

Here the movement has not been continuous, as the leg has not moved at the same time as the torso.

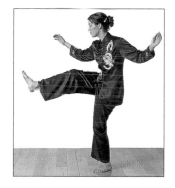

You will probably need help to co-ordinate your movements correctly.

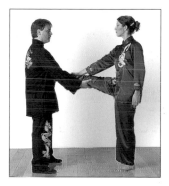

Eventually you will find that flowing movement comes naturally.

(8) UNITE THE MIND (INTENT) WITH THE BODY (FRAME)

Let us go back and see how our soldiers are faring. They are looking very much improved. They are all working together and the whole army looks and feels better. Now they no longer feel like a collection of parts, but feel instead like a co-ordinated group.

The truth, however, is slightly different. They look good and feel good, but if they actually meet another army they will be in trouble. The reason for this is that whilst being excellent at marching, they have little or no idea of what to do when they meet the enemy.

This would be similar to the Tai Chi student who can exercise the moves, but has no true understanding of them, or what they are used for. Tai Chi was invented and evolved as a martial art. If the Tai Chi student understands the moves, they can use the intent of the mind to allow Chi to flow.

Without the intent, the moves become little more than waving the arms and legs. This may be enough for a simple keep-fit exercise, but if you want the benefits that Tai Chi has to offer you must use the mind and the intent.

When you can use intent properly, energy will flow. You now have the possibility of using Chi for healing if that is one of your aims.

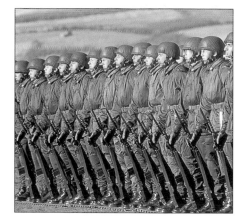

An army needs to have a balance between the physical unity of the soldiers, and their awareness and readiness for battle.

(9) USE MIND AND NOT FORCE

Tai Chi is classified by many as a 'soft' or 'internal' martial art. The meaning of 'soft' in this context relates to how you hold your muscles. The 'hard' or 'external' martial arts generally use techniques that employ strength or tension in the muscles. With 'internal' martial arts, power is a requirement, but not through muscular strength alone.

This is one feature of Tai Chi that is frequently not understood. Many Tai Chi students learn how to be soft, but they do not actually generate any power.

The reason that little or no power has been generated is that they have not understood the use of mind or 'intent'. Energy cannot flow without intent. Without intent, the Tai Chi will not be complete.

The reason that we have to be soft is to allow our energy meridians to become relaxed. Energy flows through the body via a system of channels or 'meridians'. If the body becomes tense, the flow is restricted. Softness and relaxation allow the maximum energy to travel through the body.

With Tai Chi at this level, it is the intent that is being moved rather than simply the body. This is how we move the mind and not the body for the Ninth Essence.

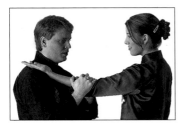

Unlike other martial arts, Tai Chi does not rely on muscular strength.

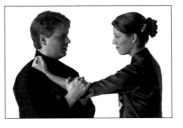

Rather, Tai Chi uses the flow of Energy to create 'intent' which increases power.

(10) SEEK STILLNESS WITHIN MOTION AND MOTION WITHIN STILLNESS.

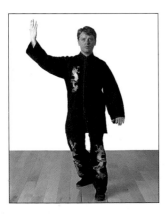

Achieving stillness is an important part of Tai Chi practice.

The Tenth Essence involves quite a high level of meditation. When one progresses into these realms of the mind and body, words cannot convey the whole of our experience (remember our original definition of Tai Chi). You will find that when people do try and convey these experiences, the descriptions are textured by their individual personalities.

However, the Tenth Essence does need some sort of definition if you are ever going to understand it for yourself. How can you go on a journey if you do not define some sort of reason for the journey and final destination?

Explanations usually come when you least expect them. Talking to others, listening to music or watching a film can all suddenly provide you with another explanation. A particularly good analogy for the Tenth Essence comes from a film. The heroine of the film is a basketball coach whose team is having problems with their shooting.

She tells the team that whenever they have possession of the ball, they are allowing themselves to become distracted by other team and the spectators. What they need to do in this situation is to be able to stop, take a breath and shoot.

In practical terms, however, this is not possible. Basketball is a fast game, the coach tells her team, and if a player were to stop even for a second, the defenders would stop them from attacking. The players needed to be able to find that calm even during the height of the action so that they can shoot. In other words, they needed to find stillness within motion. This analogy makes the martial arts application of the Essence very obvious.

When stillness within motion is found, the inner body will have the feeling of extension and creation of energy. This is how you will find motion within stillness and be able to complete the Tenth Essence.

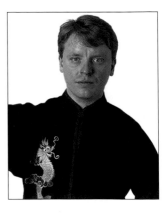

Combining motion and stillness is the key to successfully completing the Ten Essences.

Before practising Tai Chi it is essential to do some warm-up exercises. The warm-up sequences following serves several different purposes. Exercises one to eight are generally intended to get the blood and Chi flowing throughout the system. The stretches can open up meridians and the rotations are designed to help release joints that may become tense.

Exercise number nine is a very powerful energy-building exercise. These sorts of exercises are frequently called Chi Gung or Quigong. Chi Gung should be a part of every serious Tai Chi exercise routine. The standing exercise shown here is very simple, but it definitely works. Try it for a couple of weeks and see if you disagree.

The final exercise is probably one of the most valuable. It is a simple meditation that teaches you how to relax the body and mind. While you can do this through sleep, meditation allows you to develop a systematic way of relaxing the body and mind.

WARM UP EXERCISE 1 LEARNING TO STAND

Shaking and breathing is a simple way to relax the body and stimulate the flow of Chi. It also teaches you how to move the intent through your body.

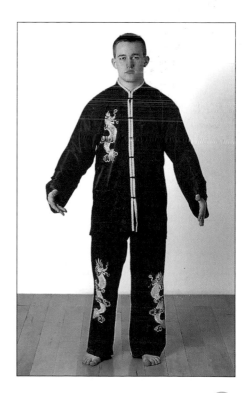

Stand in a relaxed position. Lift up your head and pull your shoulders down. Let your back become slightly rounded so that your chest becomes soft. Your feet should be shoulder-width apart and parallel. Your waist should be relaxed so that you can feel an equal distribution of weight in your feet. Have your legs straight but do not lock your knees. This will be the starting position for many of the Tai Chi warm up exercises and is actually used as the start of the form. This is called the Wu Chi posture.

Close your mouth and start to breathe softly through your nose. Allow your breathing to sink by making sure that when you breathe in, your stomach moves out and when you breath out, your stomach goes in.

This sort of breathing is fundamental to Tai Chi and all Tai Chi exercises. Do not be disappointed if it seems difficult at first or that you keep forgetting it. After some practice you will find that you will do it almost instinctively.

SHAKING

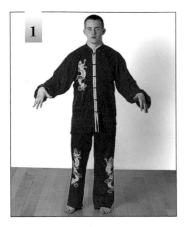

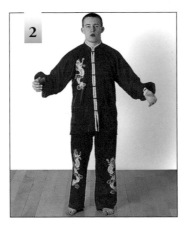

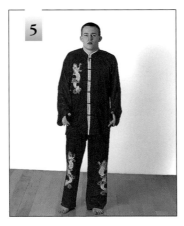

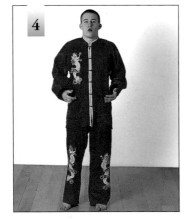

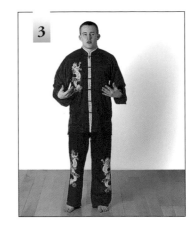

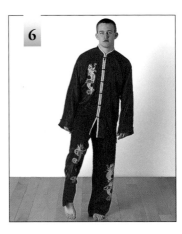

Start in the Wu Chi posture. Begin by shaking your fingertips. Imagine that Energy travelling to your fingertips. Feel each of your fingertips fill with Energy. (1)

When you can 'feel into' each of your finger tips, move your attention up into the first joint. Imagine that as you breathe Chi in through your lungs, the joint becomes more relaxed. Continue for all of the joints in your hand, working inwards from fingertips to wrist. Your hands should feel more relaxed. (2-3)

Carry on with the exercise, gradually moving attention from your wrist to your forearm and elbow. Allow your elbow to loosen, and start to move the biceps and triceps at the top of your arm. (4)

Finish by shaking your shoulders up and down, letting your arms hang free. (5)

Allow the movement to gradually slow down and stop.

Put your weight onto your left leg and start to shake the toes of your right leg. Now move the intent through your toes, foot, ankle, lower leg, knee and thigh. You will also find that this is good exercise for balancing on the standing leg. (6) Repeat the exercise for your left leg.

This exercise is quite easy to do, and warms the body up well. It is therefore worthwhile to spend a good five or ten minutes shaking and loosening up.

WARM UP EXERCISE 2 NECK ROTATIONS

Tension in the neck can cause Chi stagnation that may lead to headaches. Neck rotations free your neck, allowing better flow of Chi.

When performing any of these exercises, it is important to 'listen' to your body. If an exercise is painful, you should either ease off on the exercise, or miss it out completely. This is especially true with neck rotations, because the neck is a very delicate joint.

Start by standing in the Wu Chi position. Lift the crown of your head slightly to extend through your neck. Do not strain. Look upward. (1)

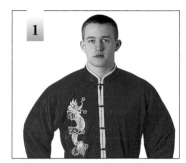

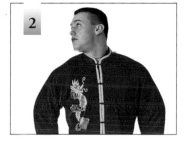 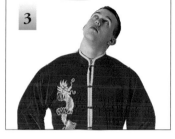 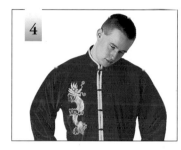 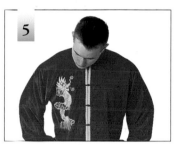

Imagine that you are drawing a circle with your eyes. Move your head around in a circle to try and make the biggest circle that you can with your eyes. Make the movement slow, to avoid pulling your neck and also to allow you to co-ordinate your breathing. (2-5)

When you feel your neck has become looser, stop and repeat in the opposite direction. Do not be alarmed if you hear a crackling noise – this is partly caused by the release of tension.

This exercise is done with your back straight and shoulders down. A common error is to try and make the biggest circle possible by moving your back with your neck

WARM UP EXERCISE 3 SHOULDER ROTATIONS

Your shoulders are very sensitive to energy changes within the body. Relaxed shoulders will have a positive effect upon the rest of the body.

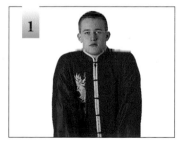 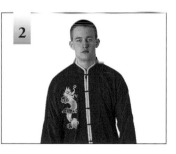 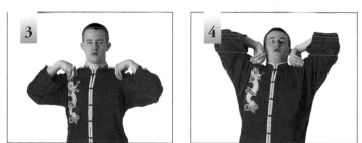

Start by standing in the Wu Chi position. On an inward breath, lift your shoulders. Time the lifting of your shoulders to be synchronous with your inward breath. (1)

When your lungs are full and your shoulders are at their maximum, slowly allow the breath out and let your shoulders descend. (2)

Alternatively, place your knuckles at your collarbones and rotate your elbows and shoulders in this position. (3-4)

Keep your back straight and your head up. Do not allow your knees to lock. You should feel the movement throughout the whole of your body, rather than just within your shoulders. Try to make the same amount of repetitions in both directions of rotation.

WARM UP EXERCISE 4 WAIST ROTATION

In Tai Chi, the waist must be free to move. This exercise also massages the kidneys and important energy points for the kidneys.

Start by standing in the Wu Chi position. Place the palms of your hands on your kidneys. Start to make small circles with your waist. The circles should start small, but increase in size. Your waist will be moving in an outward spiral. Keep your breathing relaxed. Do not overstretch and keep your feet flat on the floor. (1-3)

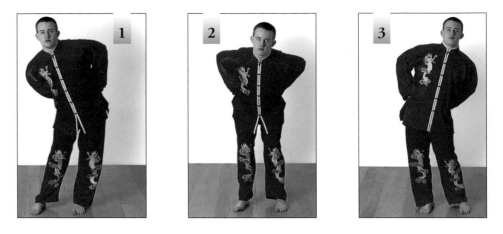

When you have come to the rest position, repeat the waist rotations in the other direction. Repeat the same amount of rotations in both directions. Beginners should be able to perform fifteen to twenty rotations. More advanced students should be setting their own limits.

WARM UP EXERCISE 5 MOVING THE WAIST AND SWINGING THE ARMS

This exercise invigorates the flow of Chi throughout the whole body and teaches you how to issue movement from the Tan Tien.

Stand in the Wu Chi posture. Oscillate your waist to the left and the right. Keep your body straight and the arms relaxed. Gradually build up speed. Do not try to simply swing your arms otherwise you will miss the point of the exercise. In the beginning your arms should swing around your waist. This gives a massage to your lower abdomen and the kidney area of your back. (1-2)

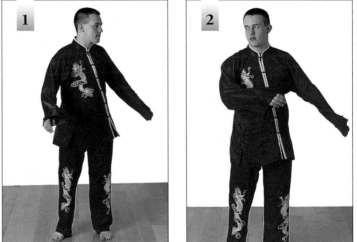

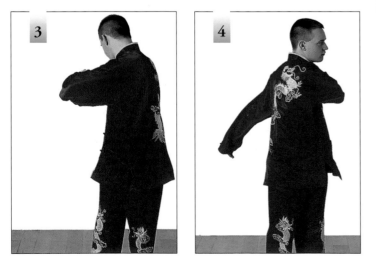

When you have trained your body further, you can use the exercise to massage your torso and neck. Do this simply by swinging your arms higher. You can throw your hand over your shoulder or work higher with your neck if you desire. Do not do this too hard, especially when massaging the neck or you may hurt yourself. Be sure to keep your shoulders down even if you are working high on the body. (3-4)

When you have had enough, let your waist momentum gradually slow down and stop. Do not try to stop suddenly because this can lead to injury. Try to keep your feet rooted into the floor during the exercise. If you can keep your feet stationary, it will improve your 'Tai Chi Root'

WARM UP EXERCISE 6 KNEE ROTATIONS

Keeping your knees healthy and loose will help to prevent arthritis. Do not attempt this exercise if you have any problems with your knees. If the exercise causes discomfort, do not continue.

This is the only physical exercise in this sequence that does not start in the Wu Chi position. Stand with both feet together, ankles touching. Bend your knees slightly and reach down to rest the palms of your hands on your kneecaps. The exercise is performed with feet flat on the floor.

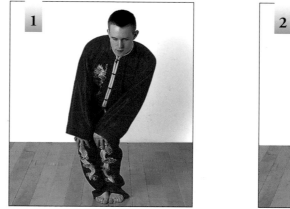

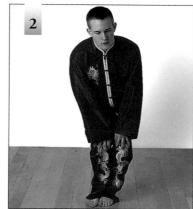

Make small circles with your knees. Allow the circles to gradually increase in size. Do not try to make the knee circles too large as this can strain your knee. (1-2)

When you have made several circles in one direction, slow down and stop. Then repeat the exercise a similar number of times in the opposite direction.

When you first try this exercise, keep the number of knee rotations low. When you have learned how your knee performs with the exercise and gained experience of it, you can increase the amount of rotations.

WARM UP EXERCISE 7 ANKLE ROTATIONS

Tension in the ankle joint will cause your movement to be less grounded. Rotations of the ankle can help release the tension and enhance the feeling of grounding.

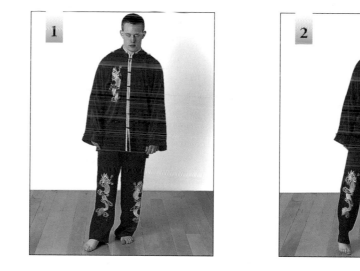

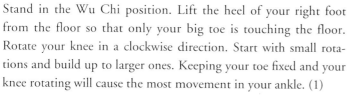

Stand in the Wu Chi position. Lift the heel of your right foot from the floor so that only your big toe is touching the floor. Rotate your knee in a clockwise direction. Start with small rotations and build up to larger ones. Keeping your toe fixed and your knee rotating will cause the most movement in your ankle. (1)

After ten to twenty rotations, slow down to a stop. Repeat with an anti-clockwise rotation of the knee (2), and then on your other leg. After you have completed the exercise, give your legs a good shake to loosen them up again.

WARM UP EXERCISE 8 LEG STRETCHES

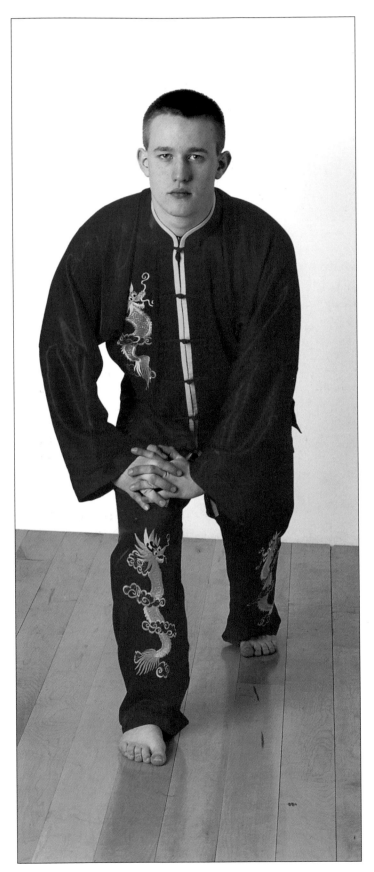

Stretching improves flexibility and helps the circulation of blood and the lymphatic system.

In this warm-up sequence there is one simple leg stretch. You may wish to investigate stretches from other martial arts, Yoga or sports exercises.

The three most important features of any stretching exercises are:

1) The body should be warmed up. Under no circumstances should you try to perform any stretching routine without warming up first.

2) Take your time If you are not quite as supple as you think you should be, there is a temptation to try and stretch too hard.

(3) Breathe. This may seem like trivial advice, but a very common mistake is to hold your breath during stretches. Keep your breathing deep and relaxed.

If a stretch causes pain, you are either trying to stretch too far or an injury is limiting the stretch. In either case the pain is a warning to stop or ease off.

Stand in the Wu Chi position. Slide your left leg straight back, and bend your right knee. Rest both hands on your right knee. The intensity of the stretch is determined by how far back you move your left leg. For the best stretch, keep the toes of your left foot pointing as far forward as possible.

Take a deep breath in. On the outward breath, push forward with your right knee. You will feel the stretch working along the back of your leg if you are performing it correctly. If your left heel lifts you are trying to stretch too far. Adjust so that you have a shorter stance.

On the inward breath, relax the stance so that the stretch relaxes. Let your knee move back and your body rise.

Repeat the stretch for ten breaths, then switch legs.

WARM UP EXERCISE 9 STANDING EXERCISES

Standing exercises are very good for increasing leg strength. They also set up the body requirements for Tai Chi and increase the Energy level.

Wu Chi Position

The foundation of the standing exercise is the Wu Chi position. It is worthwhile revisiting the Wu Chi Position before carrying on to the next position.

Relax your mind and still your internal dialogue. You may have found that simply standing in the position was difficult to maintain. There is nothing wrong with this. In many ways this can be an advantage, because you now know something that you need to work on for good Tai Chi.

You may find that quieting your mind is the most difficult part. You need to be able to let go of the other things in our lives for a time to let your body relax. If you can learn how to let go of everything for long enough to stand in the Wu Chi position for ten to fifteen minutes, you will be ready to start working on the next level — Standing Like a Tree.

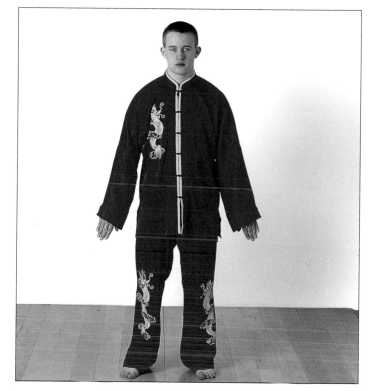

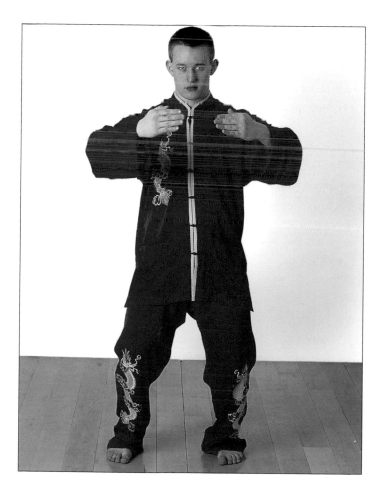

Standing Like a Tree

Part of the exercise is to imagine that your feet are extending into the floor, like tree roots. If your legs are well rooted, then you can use them to exert power. Great physical and mental stamina is developed with this exercise.

This position is physically more demanding than the last. At first, it will be difficult to maintain for any period of time. Allow slow but gradual progress. When you have been patient enough to be able to hold it for ten to fifteen minutes, you will have made such dramatic changes to yourself that you will wish that you had started the exercises years ago.

Start by standing in the familiar Wu Chi position. Bend your knees slightly to lower your torso. Keep your head, back and waist in alignment. Keep your weight equally distributed in your feet. Lift your arms in front of your chest. They should be lower than your shoulders and relaxed. Keep a gap under your armpit and point your elbows down, palms of your hands facing towards you.

The position may feel difficult at first, but stick with it. Many so-called 'muscle men' cannot hold the position while people three times their age are quite relaxed in the position. The difference is to do with internal strength, and this is your chance to cultivate it.

WARM UP EXERCISE 10 QUIET MEDITATION

During meditation blood pressure drops, the pulse slows down, the brain relaxes and stress hormones subside.

Meditation is better classified as a 'warming-down' exercise than a warming-up exercise. It is helpful to finish a Tai Chi session with ten to fifteen minutes of quiet meditation. This allows you time to cool down and relax after a training session. Meditation need not, however, be restricted to when you have been practising Tai Chi. It can be included during any part of your day. The following meditation procedure is quite simple and can be quite effective.

The meditation can be done in either a sitting or lying position. Sitting has an advantage over lying, as you are less likely to fall asleep. The difficulty with sitting meditation is that you need to keep your back straight, just as if you are in the Wu Chi position.

Choose the correct environment. Make sure you are in a well-ventilated room with plenty of fresh air. Keep warm and switch on the answerphone if you have one. Try to minimise any disturbances for the next twenty minutes or so. You may enjoy burning essential oils or listening to soft music. This can enhance the mood for meditation.

Close your eyes and relax. Have your mouth gently closed (do not clench your jaw). Breathe through your nose. Focus your mind on your breathing and let it become soft and deep. Spend a few minutes simply focussing your attention on your breathing, to allow it to become soft and regular.

Relax the muscles and skin on your forehead. Imagine that every time you breathe out, the tension is just falling away. Do the same for your eyes and the muscles of your face.

Work down through your body relaxing your neck, shoulders, arms, chest, abdomen, waist, thighs, knees, ankles and feet.

When you reach your feet, pause and bring your attention back to your breathing. Make sure it is still relaxed, deep and regular.

Now return to your forehead. Instead of relaxing the outer skin and muscles, work slightly deeper within your body. Every time you go through your body you are relaxing it with the intent of your mind. This allows you to 'peel off' layers of tension rather like the layers of an onion.

There is no time limit on this meditation exercise. If you are worried about falling asleep and missing an appointment, then set an alarm clock.

Many people appreciate the benefits of meditation, but believe they do not have enough time to do it. If you are more relaxed, you will be more efficient and healthier, so it is always worth making time for meditation.

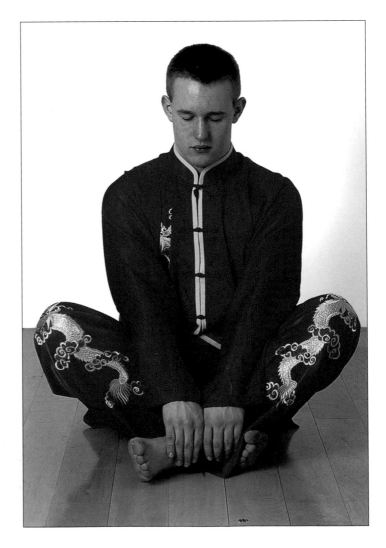

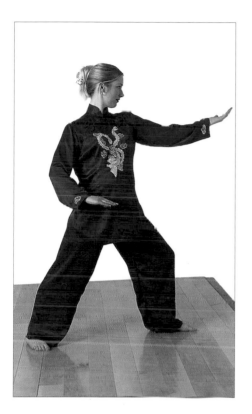

The Tai Chi form is made up of a series of flowing movements.

Martial arts can be as varied with their strategies and movements as different styles of music. Some are hard, some are soft. Some emphasise training at high speed, others prefer slower training. Some work close to the body, others work further away. Some can work with kicks and punches; others may emphasise joint locks. In nearly every style of martial art, however, part of the teaching will be set aside for learning a sequence or pattern of movements.

In Tai Chi, these sequences of movements are generally called 'forms'. The Tai Chi forms were invented by the Masters of the styles, to teach students the full syllabus of movements within that style. When you can perform the movements of a form, you will have reached a level of understanding of that style.

In the beginning, the movement may feel very clumsy. Eventually, you finish learning the form that you have chosen. You will now need to practice the whole form on your own as often as possible. An instructor will still be needed to make corrections, but the main work will be done yourself.

Greater depth is added to the form by learning two-person routines. Applications can be studied in more depth and practised with training partners. This will give you more understanding of the movements in the form.

Do not try to reach too far too soon. When you first learn how to drive, you do not head straight for the racetracks. Tai Chi is the same — take it in small steps and you will have the chequered flag before you know it.

For each movement in the form, a two-person application is illustrated.

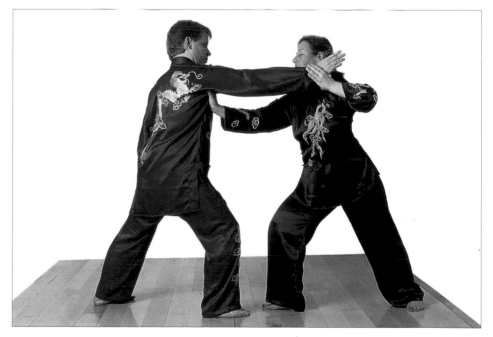

APPLICATIONS

For each Tai Chi posture described, there is a brief description of a martial arts application. For consistency, the person performing the Tai Chi move is always shown in black, while the opponent is seen in different colours. The postures are very versatile. For each application shown, there are several more possible.

THE SIMPLIFIED TAI CHI FORM

The Simplified Tai Chi Form consists of different postures, drawn together in a sequence. The sequence can be divided into four individual sections. This helps to break it into 'bite-size chunks', which can help when first learning the sequence. When you have mastered the sequence, you will no longer be concerned with individual sections. You will work with the flow of the moves.

    The sequence of the Simplified Tai Chi form is listed here. Some of the earlier moves repeat themselves, so the number of repeats is also with the sequence.

Section 1
Opening form
Parting the Wild Horse's Mane (repeat 3 times)
White Crane Spreads its Wings
Brush Knee and Twist Step (repeat 3 times)
Hand Strums the Lute

Section 2
Step Back and Repulse the Monkey (repeat 4 times)
Grasp the Sparrow's Tail (left side)
Grasp the Sparrow's Tail (right side)
Single Whip
Wave Hands like Clouds (repeat 3 times)
Single Whip

Section 3
High Pat on Horse
Turn and Kick with Right Heel
Strike opponents Ears with Both Fists
Turn and Kick with Left Heel
Snake Creeps Down (left side)
Golden Rooster Stand on One Leg (right side)
Snake Creeps Down (left side)
Golden Rooster Stand on One Leg (left side)
Snake Creeps Down (right side)

Section 4
Fair Lady Works at Shuttles
Needle at the Sea Bottom
Fan through Back
Turn around, Parry, Block and Punch
Apparent Close-up
Closing Form

THE STANCES

In Yang style Tai Chi there are only four stances. These are:

(1) Parallel Stance. Used in the opening form, closing form and *Waving Hands like Clouds.*

(2) Bow Stance. Used in *Parting the Wild Horse's Mane, Brush Knee and Twist Step, Grasp the Sparrow's Tail, Single Whip, Fair Lady Works Shuttles, Fan through the Back, Parry, Block and Punch* and *Apparent Close-up.*

(3) Empty Stance. Used in *White Crane Spreads its Wings, Strum the Lute, Repulse the Monkey, High Pat on Horse, Kicks, Golden Rooster stands on One Leg* and *Needle at the Sea Bottom.*

(4) Drop Stance. Used only with *Snake Creeps Down.*

If you find that you are standing in any other stance during the form, then it is wrong and needs correcting. It is therefore essential to gain a good understanding of the postures.

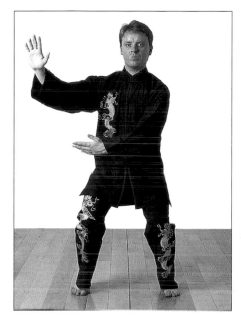

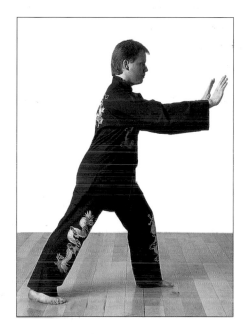

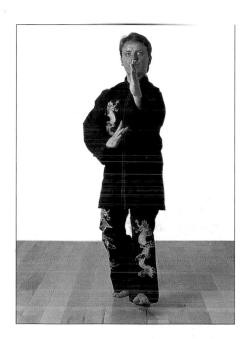

PARALLEL STANCE

This is the only stance during the whole of the form where the weight is equal in both legs. This only occurs during the opening and commencing forms. The weight is actually shifting during *Waving Hands like Clouds*, but the posture remains the same.

BOW STANCE

In the Bow Stance, the weight is approximately 70% on the front leg and 30 % on the back leg. There are two variations of the Bow Stance. One is where the torso of the body and the back leg are straight, and the other is where the torso is vertical.

EMPTY STANCE

The Empty Stance is regarded by many as the most difficult. This is because all your weight is supported entirely on your back leg.

DROP STANCE

The Drop Stance is very similar to the Bow Stance, except that your weight is on your back leg and your torso has dropped lower.

HAND POSITIONS

A simple and easy way for the beginner to judge the skill level of a person more experienced in Tai Chi is to look at the person's hands when they are practising. The reason for this is not that the hand movements are excessively complicated, rather they exactly the opposite. The shapes of the hands in Tai Chi are deceptively simple.

There are only three actual shapes for the hands in the simplified Tai Chi form. These are the open hand, fist and 'Tiger's Mouth'. If you have managed to achieve the skill level where you do not need to 'try' to remember the form, then you will be able to give more of your attention to the hands. When you no longer need to 'try' to maintain correct hands positioning, you can move your attention to another aspect of Tai Chi.

OPEN HAND (TAI CHI PALM)

During Tai Chi practice, a common mistake is to hold your hands limp (1). This stops Energy from travelling to your fingertips, making them appear lifeless. Limpness in the hand will also deny any understanding of martial applications, and therefore the intent will not be exercised. Without intent, you will not be able to feel the strength of the Energy.

Usually after being instructed not to have limp hands, the student will go to the other extreme. The hand will become very tight and exert too much force (2). This will hinder the movement and affect the blood circulation.

The correct way of holding the hand for the Tai Chi Palm is somewhere in between a limp and a tight hand. The fingers should be extended, but they should also be relaxed (3). The thumb is relaxed and quite close to the hand. This allows proper circulation of blood and Energy so the hands will feel more alive.

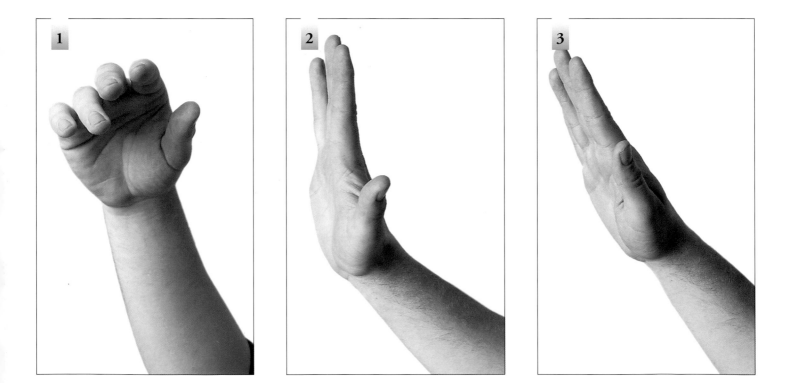

TIGER'S MOUTH

After learning the Tai Chi palm, the 'Tiger's Mouth' is easy. To make the shape for Tiger's Mouth, simply make the Tai Chi palm and move the thumb outwards. Keep the hand relaxed but extended as before. This hand shape only occurs in *Hand Strums the Lute*, at the end of Section 1.

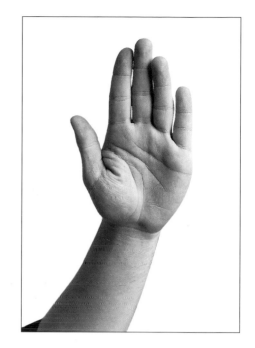

TAI CHI FIST

Fists are used quite frequently towards the latter end of the form. The fist in Tai Chi is similar to the fist used in many other martial arts, except that it is relaxed. If the fist becomes too tense, it will need correcting.

To make the Tai Chi fist, start by making the Tai Chi palm. Now roll the fingers towards the hand, so that they touch the palm. Finish the fist by bringing the thumb down over the first two fingers (1).

A common mistake is to bend the wrist when making a fist (2). The Energy to the fist should come in a straight line from the elbow. If you bend your wrist, you will simply not be able to transmit any appreciable power through the fist. Also, if you prefer to think in martial arts terms, if you were to hit anything with a fist that was bent, you would hurt your wrist.

Another common mistake is to make a 'hollow' fist (3). This is again incorrect for the style of Tai Chi studied here.

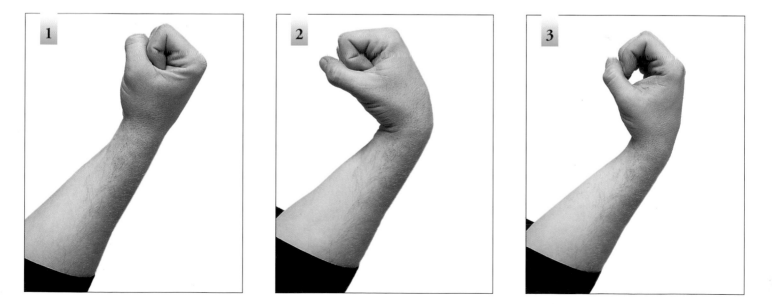

SECTION 1

(1) OPENING FORM

The opening form is symbolic of the Taoist image of the creation of the Universe. In the beginning there was the absolute void, known as Wu Chi. In this void, Energies began moving. They existed in a state of attraction and repulsion, until they gathered together to polarise in opposites. This was the beginning of Yin and Yang. When Yin and Yang are created, they create the 'Ten Thousand Things'.

THE MOVEMENT

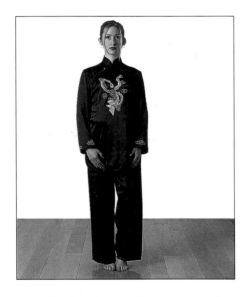

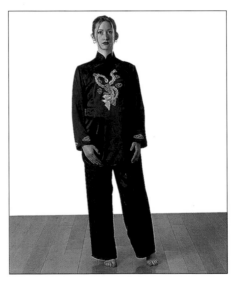

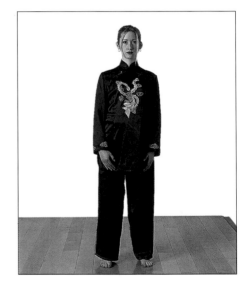

Start the form by standing with your feet together and your arms relaxed. The weight should be equally carried in both legs at this point. Without moving your body, push the right heel into the floor so that it carries more of your body weight. As your right leg carries more of the weight, it follows that your left leg will feel lighter.

As your left leg starts to feel lighter, allow your left knee to rise. When all of your body weight is carried on your right leg, it is time to step to the side with your left leg. This is done by lifting up first the heel and then the toes. When the toes have lifted, move your left foot to the left. The position should be such that when your feet are placed on the ground, they are one shoulder width apart and parallel.

Touch your toe to the floor and then your heel. Do not place your weight straight down, otherwise your step will become clumsy. When your foot is finally on the floor, adjust your weight so that is no longer all carried on your right leg but 50 % on each leg. This is the last time that the weight will be 'double weighted' in your legs before the closing form.

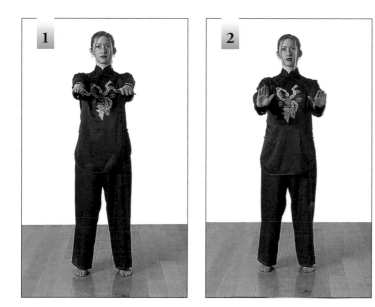

Extend your fingertips gently. On the inward breath raise them up to shoulder level. On the outward breath, lower your shoulders,

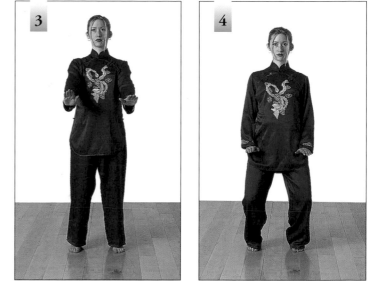

elbows, forearms and finally your hands. When your hands face the floor, sink your body slightly. (1-4)

Visualisation

Imagine that when you are raising your hands you are extending Chi through your fingertips. When you lower the body, imagine that you are pushing Energy through your feet into the floor, and forming a root.

Application

Your opponent has grabbed hold of you by the wrists. You can throw your opponent by raising your hands. For this application to work you must remain soft and visualise Energy extending past the fingertips. (1-3)

Do not try to use muscular force, as this will simply result in the strongest person winning. In Tai Chi applications, it is always assumed that your opponent is stronger than you are. This means that you have to use technique, rather than strength if you are to stand a chance.

POINTS TO WATCH OUT FOR:

- When raising and lowering your arms, keep your torso straight. Do not lean forward or back.

- Synchronise breathing with the movement. Avoid all stiffness in the movement.

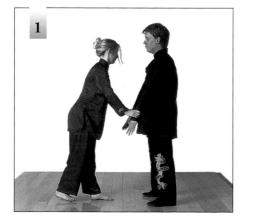

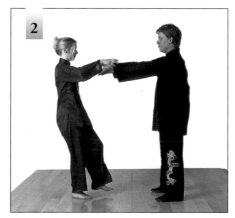

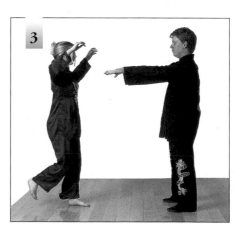

(2) PARTING THE WILD HORSE'S MANE

When trying to tame a wild horse, it is essential to stay relaxed. If you become tense or fearful, then the horse will detect it and you will not gain the upper hand.

This is true with the Tai Chi forms when used in combat. If an opponent can detect that you are afraid, then you will not gain control. It is essential to stay calm, but have strong intent.

THE MOVEMENT

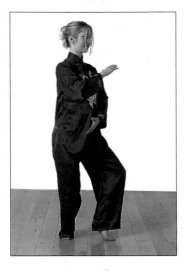 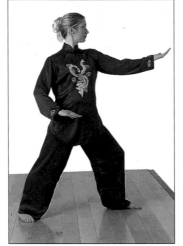 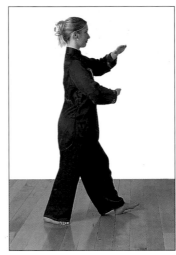 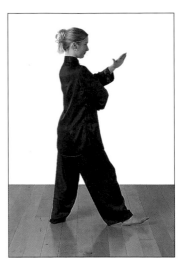

Sink your weight on to your right leg. Allow your waist to turn to the left. Lift your left heel, move your left hand down and your right hand upwards in a circular direction. Lift your left leg and place it forward and to the left, so that you can make a Bow Stance. Place your foot on the floor first with the heel and then the toe. Do not shift your weight yet.

Push your weight from your right leg to the left, so that your body will finish in the Bow Stance, with most of your weight on the front leg. Your left hand will uncoil from the lower position to the higher. Move first your shoulder, then your elbow and finally your hand. Your hand finishes facing upwards. Your right hand presses down and finishes with the fingers pointing in the direction of travel. Gaze gently over your left hand.

Shift the weight back on to your right leg. Relax your arms, but keep them in approximately the same position. Turn your waist, so that your toes turn to an angle of 45°. Push all your weight from your right leg to the left. When all your weight is carried on your left leg, step through in a straight line with your right leg. This is how you will move forward in the Bow Stance.

When your right foot is placed flat on the floor you are ready to move forward into the next Bow Stance. Shift your weight from your left leg to the right by turning your waist.

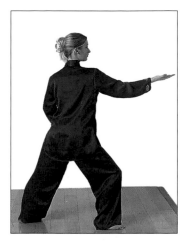

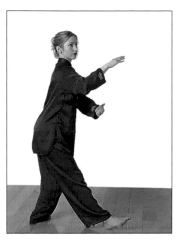

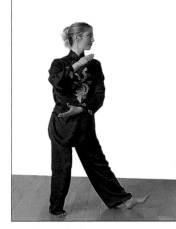

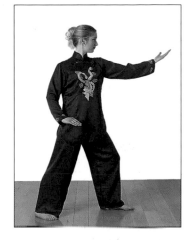

Bring your right arm up in a circular motion and press your left arm down. This completes the second part of the move.

Shift your weight from your right leg back to the left. Turn your toes out to an angle of 45°. Move your weight forward onto your right leg.

Step forward with your left leg to create another Bow Stance.

Turn your waist to push your weight from your right leg back to the left. At the same time, your left arm spirals upward and your right arm presses down.

Visualisation

Imagine that as your leading hand moves out, you are extending Chi through your shoulder, elbow and finally your hand. Try to feel a connection between your left and right hand. Imagine that when they move apart, Energy is being split or stretched.

Application

Move a leg behind your opponent's knees. You then extend into the posture and push your opponent over your leg. (1–3)

This is an example of a technique uncoiling from the centre. If you were to try to move just your hand to the position it would be easy to stop. If you move your shoulder first, then your elbow and finally your hand, it will be more difficult to stop. This also gives the effect of a triple strike, rather than a single one.

POINTS TO WATCH OUT FOR:

- Keep your head and torso straight at all times. If you tip either way, then balancing will be more difficult, and the move will become heavy. Keep your arms relaxed.

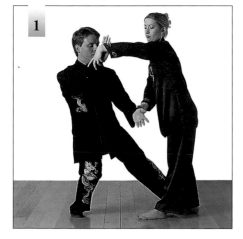

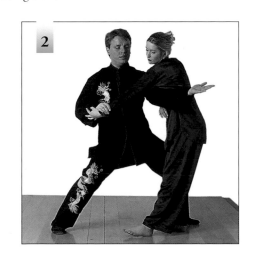

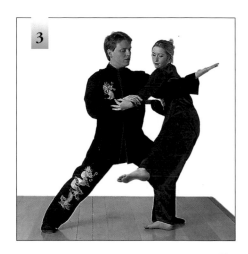

(3) WHITE CRANE SPREADS ITS WINGS

The image of the White Crane is a bird drying its wings in the sun. This is a symbol of receiving Energy from the heavens.

THE MOVEMENT

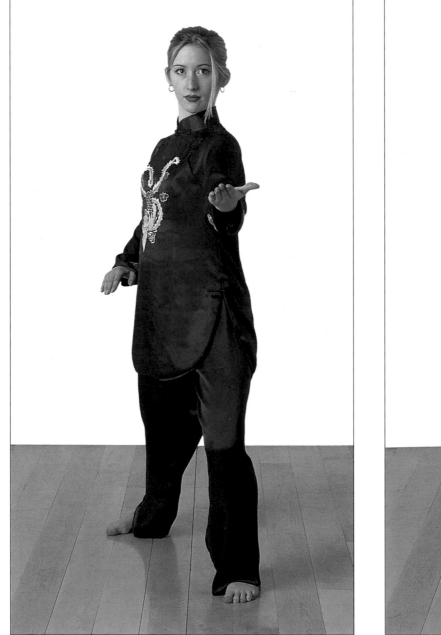

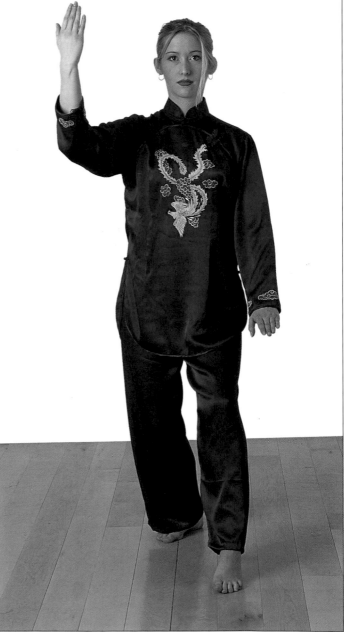

Relax both arms. Take half a step forward by sinking all your weight on to your left leg.

As you move forward, your forearms turn over so that your hands face one another.

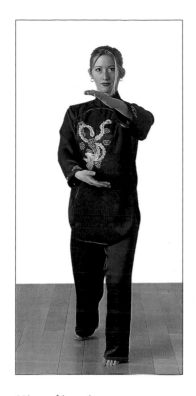

Shift your weight back onto your right leg. Simultaneously, your hands move towards each other. Lift your left heel.

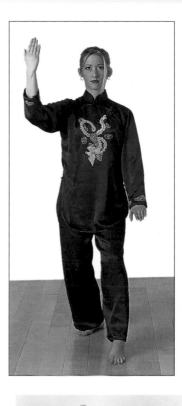

Adjust your left foot by picking it up and moving it in line with your right heel. The heel should be slightly lifted from the floor. This will put you into the Empty Stance. As your foot adjusts, raise your right arm and lower the left. The palm of your right hand should be facing towards you.

Visualisation

Imagine that as you are moving your arms up and down they are creating a shield of protective Chi around you. When you are in the final position of the move, draw Energy in from the heavens with your right hand and from the earth with your left hand.

Application

Your opponent tries to punch you. Block down with your left hand and raise your right hand to your opponent's elbow. This can then be used as a block followed by an arm-locking technique. If the move is extended into its final posture, the opponent will be thrown. (1-3)

If your Empty Stance is weak, the technique will be weak, and you will go off balance easily. As your legs get stronger, the arm movements will become easier.

POINTS TO WATCH OUT FOR:

- The body should move as a whole. Do not thrust the chest forward, and keep the shoulders down.

- If it is difficult to keep the shoulders down in the final position, do not raise the right hand as high.

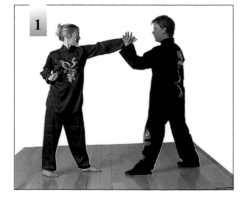

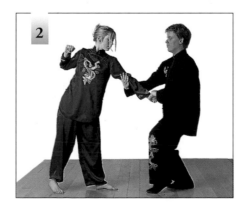

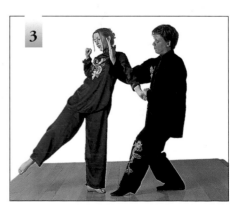

(4) BRUSH KNEE AND TWIST STEP

To execute this move properly, you must pay detailed attention to the timing of your hands and feet. When you have gained control of the timing for this move, it is easier to apply it to other moves.

THE MOVEMENT

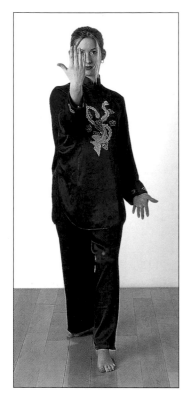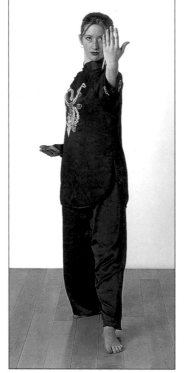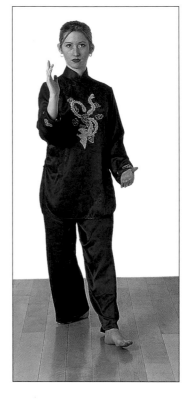

From the *White Crane Spreads its Wings* posture, your right hand moves across to guard your face, and your left hand turns over.

Turn your waist back to the right. Let your right arm move down in an arc. As your right arm moves down, your left arm moves up to protect your face again. Step out with your left leg to get ready for the Bow Stance.

To make the Bow Stance, your foot has to move forward and to the left. Simultaneous with the moving of your foot, your arms move. Your left forearm will press down, as if blocking a punch. Your right arm moves around radially to a position near to your head.

This is preparation for the actual push. Your back should be straight and all your weight carried on your right leg.

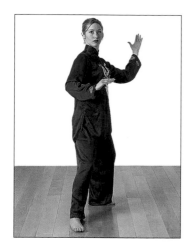 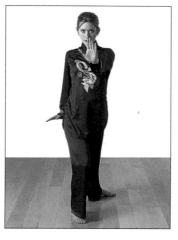 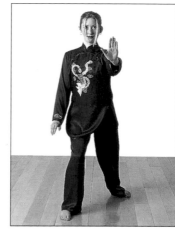 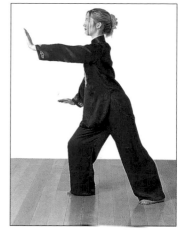

For the push, the movement is powered by pushing the weight from your left leg to the right.

As your weight transfers from your left leg to the right, your left hand performs the push and your right hand pushes past your knee.

All of the pushes in the sequence are performed in this way, whether the push is with one or two hands, and if the hand is closed to become a fist.

Shift your bodyweight on to your left leg. When your left leg has control of your weight, your right leg can step forward into the Bow Stance. As your right leg moves forward, press down with your right forearm and raise your left hand

Push your weight from your left leg to the right. As your weight moves forward, the push is performed with your left hand and your right arm brushes past your right knee. – side view)

Visualisation

Imagine that when you are doing the push, energy is being pushed through the centre of your palm. When you are stepping forward to prepare for the push, you are gathering Energy for a push.

POINTS TO WATCH OUT FOR:

- Your torso should be held vertical at all times except for the final execution of the push, where your back lines up with your back leg. Do not lock your arms. Keep your shoulders level for the final push.

Application

If your opponent tries to strike with the left hand, you can re-direct the attack with your left hand. If the deflection is soft, your opponent will keep moving forward, becoming off-balance. This is then the opportunity for the push to knock them over. (1-3)

The block here is frequently mistaken for a hard block that will stop the opponent in his tracks. The technique is better thought of as re-directing, as you use your opponent's Energy against himself.

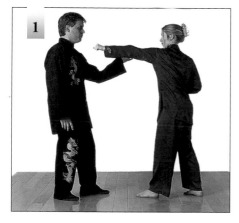 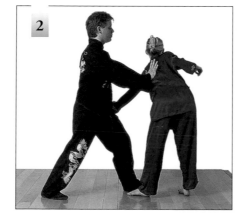 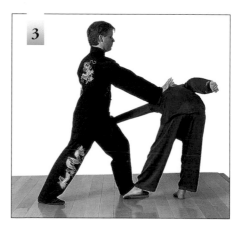

(5) HAND STRUMS THE LUTE

The significance of playing a musical instrument is to represent the idea of 'playing your own tune'. When playing your own tune you should feel a sense of inner joyfulness, being happy with what you are.

THE MOVEMENT

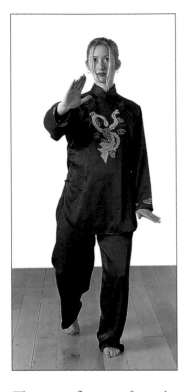 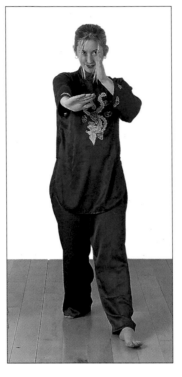 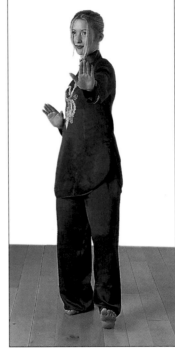 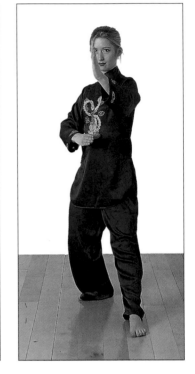

The move flows on from the last *Brush Knee and Twist Step.* Your left leg should be forward, and your right arm extended. Start the movement by leading with your waist, and shifting forward by half a step. Your body weight will first have to transfer to your left leg. This will allow you to lift your right foot from the floor. (Remember to pick up first the heel and then the toes).

You need to be firm on your left leg, otherwise it is easy to lose balance. At this moment, your arms should be relaxed — all the work is done with your legs. When your right foot has moved forward slightly, place it firmly on the floor. Your body weight will then transfer back onto your right leg.

Extend your left foot forward into the Empty Stance. The heel of your left foot will be touching the floor, with the toes slightly raised. Do not raise your toes too high, otherwise your ankle will become tense.

As your waist moves forward, your arms will extend. As your body starts to sink onto your right leg, your hands will move in an arc towards your body. The movement finishes when your weight has sunk down onto your right leg. Your left hand will be in the Tai Chi palm, with fingers pointing up and elbow pointing downwards. Your right hand will be lower than the left. It will be in the 'Tiger's Mouth' shape, with thumb extended.

Visualisation

When your hands are circling in front of your body, imagine that you are drawing Energy to your body. When you reach the final position, imagine that the fingers of your left hand extend up to the heavens. This allows you to extend your Energy and make a strong move.

Application

If a push had been done from the last move, *Brush Knee and Twist Step*, there is always the chance that it may not hit the target. In a real situation, if your opponent actually did miss, there is a good chance that he or she may try to grab your hand. This is made likely by the fact that your hand is extended towards the opponent. (1-3)

In Tai Chi, you do not fight force with force, so you would not try to snatch your hand back. Instead, you would take half a step forward. This would make your opponent think they had beaten you, and they would relax. It is at this moment that you sink your weight onto your right leg again, sink your left elbow and raise your left fingers.

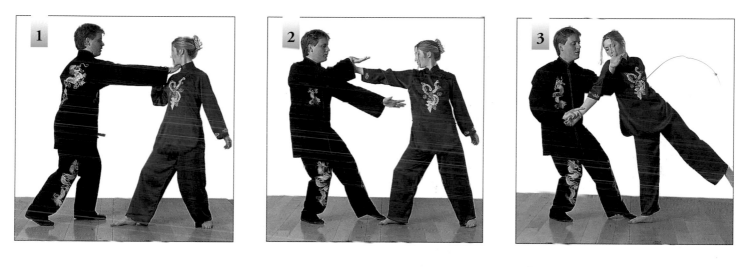

SECTION 2

When you have reached this point in your practice, you will have already started to learn the basics of Tai Chi.

You will know all the basic stances and how to move forward in the Bow Stance. The stances will not be perfect yet, and the movement will sometimes be slightly off-balance. This does not matter because they are things that you know about and you are working on them.

You may feel that from the limited amount that you have already learned, you can centre yourself better. This is a feeling that will increase as you become more proficient. Some students will be starting to get a good feeling for Energy, but do not worry if that has not happened yet — it will.

When you can manage to do the whole of Section 1, you will be ready to move onto the next section. Although it can be tempting at this stage to try some of the more difficult-looking moves in Section 3, you will find learning easier if you progress through the sections in order.. You will find that if you build a strong foundation to your Tai Chi, that the more difficult-looking moves are not as difficult as they looked at first.

When you read the introduction to this book, did you actually try to write down your own definition of Tai Chi? If you did, this is one of the points where it can pay dividends. Try repeating the exercise again. Define in your own terms what you think Tai Chi is. When you have done this, compare it to your original definition. This can make very interesting reading, because it can help you to define what you are actually getting from Tai Chi. Repeating this exercise after you have learned each section would be a worthwhile practice.

(6) STEP BACK AND REPULSE THE MONKEY

When practising Tai Chi or any other sort of meditation, it is easy to become distracted. Different thoughts seem to come into our heads almost as if it is the thoughts that are in control and not ourselves. There is a Chinese symbol for these distractions — the monkey. *Repulse the Monkey* is representative of the need to quieten our minds from the distracting 'monkey thoughts', so that we can focus our Energy on what we are doing.

The Movement

In the beginning the movement will be best executed if it is broken up into parts, as shown here. This may feel slightly mechanical, but it teaches you how to go through the individual phases of the movement correctly. Once you have gained sufficient experience you will find that the movement will automatically start to flow in an unforced way.

FIRST MOVEMENT

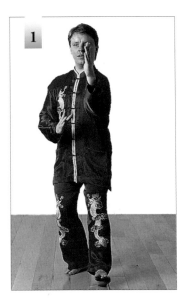

Start from the *Hand Strums the Lute* posture in Section 1. Sink your weight lower onto your right leg. This is done by keeping your right foot firmly planted on the floor, while lowering your torso slightly. Keep your back straight when sinking.

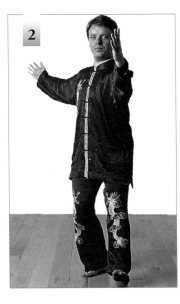

This sinking movement causes the toes on your left foot to rise slightly. As the toes rise, turn your torso to the right and open your arms. The finishing position for your arms has a similar feeling to the standing exercise – *Standing Like a Tree*. Your waist should turn to the right as your body sinks, so that it moves in a spiral.

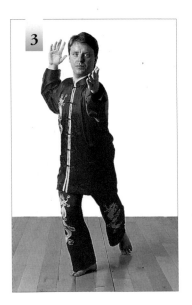

Step back with your left leg. When your left leg moves back, it travels in a straight line and the toes touch the floor first. As your left leg moves back, turn your left forearm, so that your palms are facing upwards. Synchronous with this movement, your right palm travels up in an arc to come near to your ear. There should be a straight line from your left leg through your back in this position. The toe of your left foot touches the floor.

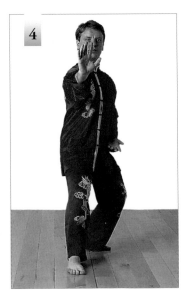

Push your weight from your right leg to the left, finishing in Empty Stance. In this version of Empty Stance your right foot is flat on the floor, but your weight is still completely supported on your left leg.

As you sink back into the Empty Stance, push your right palm outwards and pull your left elbow straight back to your torso. Your left hand finishes at belt level, facing upwards. Your right palm is extended in a push. Your body should be at a 45° angle, but your eyes will always look ahead with this move.

The second, third and fourth movements of the Repulse Monkey sequence are all repeats of the first one. The only difference between the moves is that they alternate between the left and right hand sides. The same also applies to the application.

Visualisation

Use your mind to extend Energy through your palm on the press part of the move. Feel rooted when in the Empty Stance. Imagine that Energy extends to the floor like the roots of a tree.

To keep your torso straight, imagine that your Energy is growing up from your root, like the branches of a tree.

Keep the mind clear. Do not allow any distracting thoughts — keep the Monkeys away!

SECOND MOVEMENT

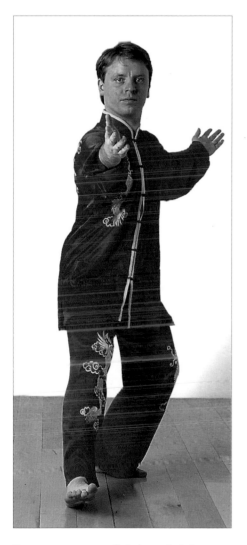

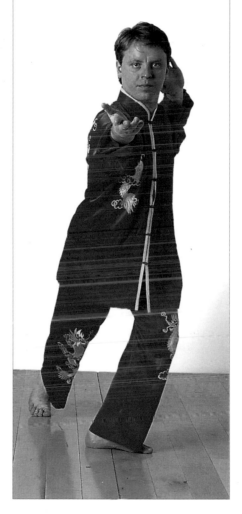

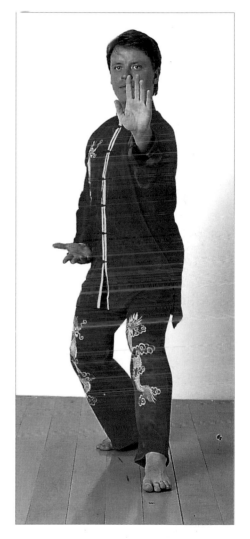

Lower your torso slightly and sink your weight onto your left leg. As your torso sinks, raise your right toes, open your left arm and turn your right forearm so that the palm faces upwards.

Step back with your right leg and touch your right toes to the floor. As your right leg travels backwards your left hand will move close to your left ear and your body will lean forward slightly.

Push your bodyweight from your left leg back onto your right leg for an Empty Stance. As your weight moves back onto your right leg, pull your right elbow back to your torso and push your left palm outwards.

THIRD MOVEMENT

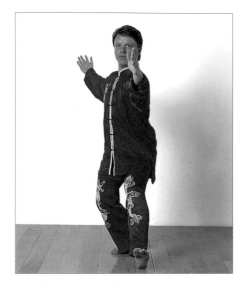 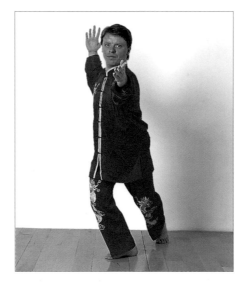 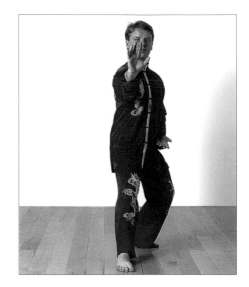

Lower your torso slightly and sink your weight onto your right leg. As your torso sinks, raise your left toes, open your right arm and turn your left forearm so that your palm faces upwards.

Step back with your left leg and touch your left toes to the floor. As your left leg travels backwards your right hand will move close to your right ear and your body will lean forward slightly.

Push your bodyweight from your right leg back onto your left leg for an empty stance. As your weight moves back onto your left leg, pull your left elbow back to your torso and push your right palm outwards.

FOURTH MOVEMENT

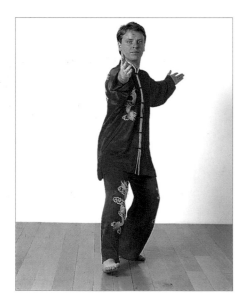 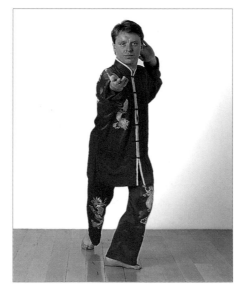 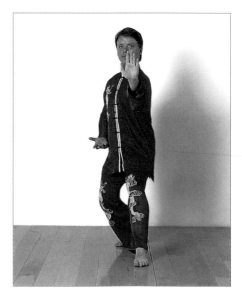

Lower your torso slightly and sink your weight onto your left leg. As your torso sinks, raise your right toes, open your left arm and turn your right forearm so that your palm faces upwards.

Step back with your right leg and touch your right toes to the floor. As your right leg travels backwards your left hand will move close to your left ear and your body will lean forward slightly.

Push your bodyweight from your left leg back onto your right leg for an Empty Stance. As your weight moves back onto your right leg, pull your right elbow back to your torso and push your left palm outwards.

APPLICATION

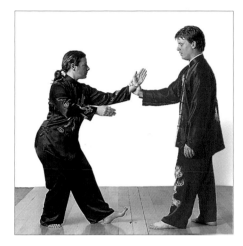 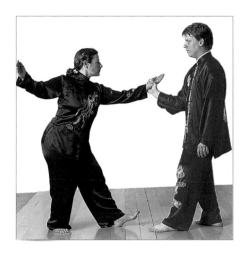 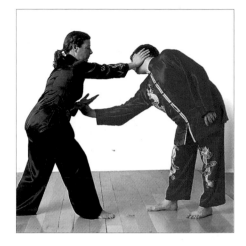

If your opponent grabs hold of your wrist, you can extend your fingertips slightly and turn the forearm over. This will cause your attacker's grip to weaken, so that you can move your opponent.

As you turn the forearm, the othr hand prepares to strike and the stepping leg moves back.

As you step back and sink, you will pull your attacker off-balance towards you. As your opponent is pulled inwards, you can strike the head or neck with the palm of the hand.

POINTS TO WATCH OUT FOR:

- It is only during the second part of the move when your foot moves back, that your body will lean forward. Try to keep your torso straight at all other parts of the move.

- Generally we are not accustomed to walking backwards. This can cause confusion with the footwork during the execution of the move. Think about using the Empty Stance, and how you are going to get into it.

- Your foot should move backwards in a straight line. Do not swing your leg out during the movement. Also be careful to avoid crossing your feet.

- Your hips can sometimes stick out when moving back. Try to avoid this possibility by being aware of it.

GRASPING THE SPARROW'S TAIL

In Chinese mythology, the sparrow brings you into your life. Grasping onto the sparrow's tail brings your spirit into the lives we live today. The lesson is that we must keep a gentle grasp onto the sparrow that brings us into life.

If we pull too hard the sparrow will not be able to take us. If we do not hold on at all we will miss the ride completely. *Grasping the Sparrow's Tail* consists of four separate moves that are bound together in a logical sequence. These four movements are Ward Off (Peng), Roll Back (Lu), Squeeze (Qi) and Press (An).

MOVEMENT

The sequence for Grasping the Sparrow's Tail is made from the four parts described earlier — Ward Off, Roll Back, Squeeze and Press. In between each of these parts there is a position that prepares you to do the move. Therefore, in total there are eight moves to the sequence. For greater clarity, each part of the sequence will be described as an individual entity. When you have grown accustomed to the four Energies, they will flow one after the other.

1. WARD OFF

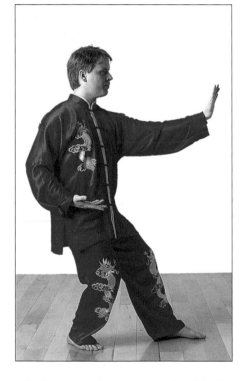 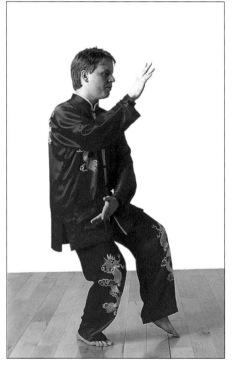 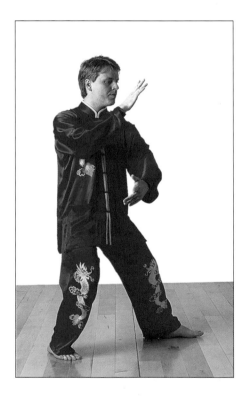

The last move that your completed in the sequence was *Repulse the Monkey.* From this position, sink your weight lower on your right leg.

As your weight sinks, your left arm moves down in an arc and your right arm rises in an arc.

When all of your weight is carried on your right leg and your position is stable, lift your left foot and step out ready for the Bow Stance. Keep your back straight and do not lean.

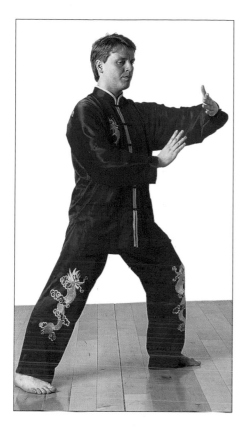

Push your weight from your right leg to the left. As your weight moves forward, raise your left forearm until it is in front of your chest with the palm turned slightly inward.

Press down with your right hand until it is below your left forearm, with the palm turned outward. It should finish between the elbow and the wrist of your left forearm.

Visualisation

In the Ward Off posture, extend Energy through the fingers of your left hand. Imagine that the fingers of the ward-off arm are extending towards infinity.

POINTS TO WATCH OUT FOR:

- Ensure that your left arm is extended but not tense. Your back leg should be straight but not locked. If your back leg is not straight, then you will not have maximised the push from it.

- In the finishing posture, your waist should be at an angle of 45° to the right.

2. ROLL BACK

Press down with your left knee to turn your waist. If your shin is vertical then your knee will not move, but your weight will shift. Use the turning of your waist to extend your arms upwards and roll your forearms. Your waist should point approximately 45° to the left. (1) Sink your weight back onto your right leg. As your weight sinks, pull your right elbow back and press your left forearm forward. The forearms rotate during the movement. (2)

Visualisation

When your arms lift, they should be very soft. This can be achieved by pressing down with your legs, so that Energy is forced downwards and your hands feel lighter.

POINTS TO WATCH OUT FOR:

- Be sure that the movement of your arms follows your waist. The movement of your arms should be well co-ordinated with your waist.

- In the final position, your left arm should be just under your right elbow. Do not bring your hands too low. Keep a gap under your armpits.

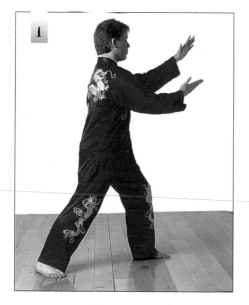

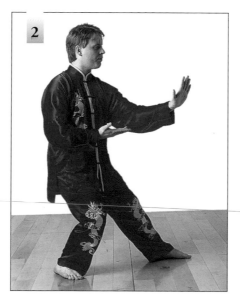

3. SQUEEZE

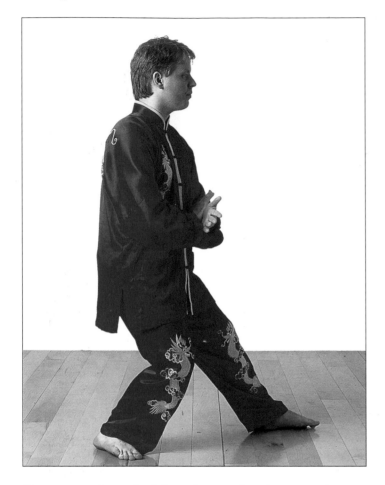 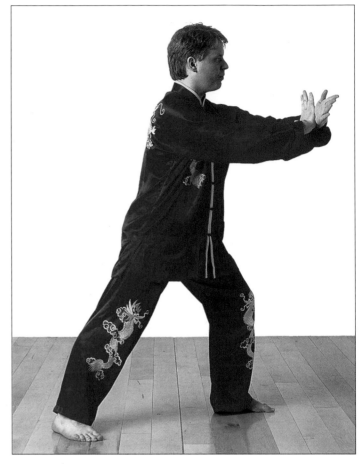

Turn your waist to the left so that you face the centre. As your waist turns, sink your torso slightly so that it spirals downwards. Lower your left arm to your abdomen. Move your right hand to touch the inside of your left forearm near to your wrist.

Push with your right leg to extend your arms forward. As your weight moves gradually forward onto your left leg, your arms extend.

Visualisation

Squeeze Energy is similar to the motion of a billiard ball. If two billiard balls are touching each other and one is hit by a third ball, the ball that was hit will transfer its kinetic energy to the ball touching it. The touching ball will then be forced to move.

Imagine that you are pressing Energy with your right hand to be transmitted through your left forearm. Extend your arms forward and push Energy towards your opponent.

POINTS TO WATCH OUT FOR:

• Do not raise your shoulders or lock your elbows for the push forward. Your left palm should stay near to your wrist for maximum strength.

• When connecting the palm to the forearm, your hand simply goes straight to your forearm. It need not follow any elaborate routes that would slow it down.

• Your arms should finish at shoulder height with elbows lower than your wrist.

4. PRESS

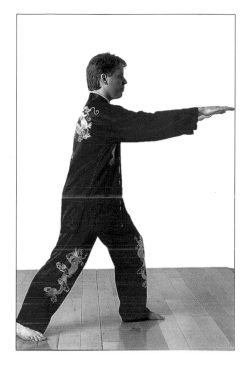

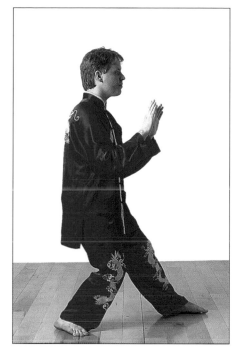

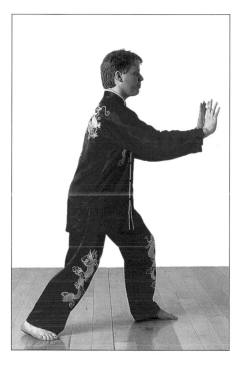

The separation of your hands is performed by turning your waist, and not just moving your hands. Your hands should finish with the distance of your forearm between the palms. Do not lock your arms hand.

Push your bodyweight from your left leg, so that it sinks onto your right leg. As your weight sinks, withdraw both of your hands in a shallow arc downwards. Make sure that when your hands have finished their journey inwards you still have a gap underneath your armpits.

Extend the push by starting it at your right heel and pushing the whole of your body forward. Your right leg and arms should be straight but not locked in the final posture. Co-ordinate the movement of your elbows with the movement of your right knee.

Visualisation

Energy travels from your hand, through a point in the centre of your palm. When your hands are moving in towards you, let your hands be very soft. Draw Energy in through the point in the palm. When your arms are extended try to feel Energy moving from that point.

When your hands move backwards and forwards, they do not follow the same line. Imagine that your fingertips are tracing the shape of a drop of water

Application

Applications for *Grasping the Sparrow's Tail* are exactly the same on both the left and right sides. To avoid unnecessary repetition, applications are detailed for the right hand side only.

POINTS TO WATCH OUT FOR:

- Keep your shoulders down and elbows pointing downwards. Do not lock your elbows for the push. Conversely, make sure that you finish the push. Your elbows should be straight in the final posture.

- When you bring your hands back to your chest, try to not try to bring them too close. If you can no longer feel a gap under your armpit when you pull your arms back, then you have pulled them in too far.

- Make sure that your fingers do not feel dead. They should be alive with Energy and intent, not loose and flaccid.

4. PRESS

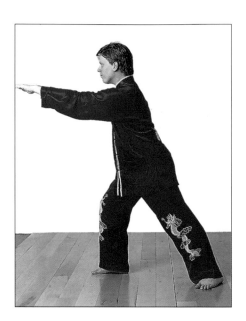

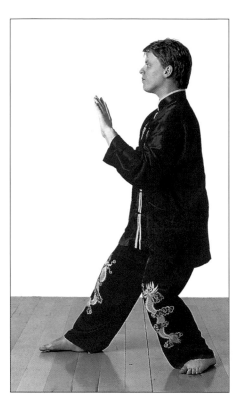

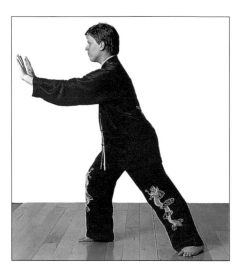

Turn your waist clockwise to separate your hands. The separation of your hands is performed by turning your waist, and not just moving your hands. Your hands should finish with the distance of your forearm between the palms. Do not lock your arms or let the hands become tight.

Push your body weight from your right leg, so that it sinks onto your rear left leg. As your weight sinks onto your left leg, withdraw both of your hands in a shallow arc downwards. Make sure that when your hands have finished their journey inwards that you still have a gap underneath your armpits.

Extend the push by starting it at your left heel and pushing the whole of your body forward. Your left leg and arms should be straight but not locked in the final posture. Co-ordinate the movement of your elbows with the movement of your left knee.

APPLICATIONS

Remember to be very careful when practising Tai Chi applications. The techniques explained are real and not just memory aids. *Grasping the Sparrow's Tail* involves extensive use of

joint locks to the elbow and shoulder. These locking techniques can cause injury if used over-zealously. Moving in a slow and relaxed manner is safer, and both partners will learn more.

WARD OFF

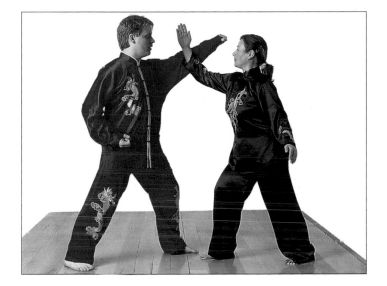

If your partner punches towards you with a left fist, raise the fingers of your right hand to block with your forearm. Do not stop moving once you have started. Move your forearm around in a circle bringing your partner's fist with it. You will need to keep your arm soft, so that you can stay in contact with your partner.

You will now have control of your partner's arm by locking the elbow. If you push the Ward Off movement it will lift your partner's shoulder which can put him or her off-balance.

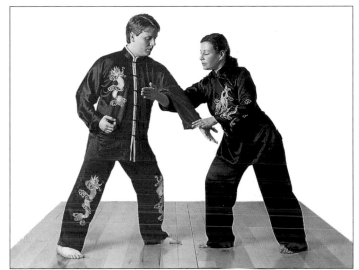

When you have brought the fist low, grab it with your left hand to gain control. While you have control of their fist with your left hand, slide your right forearm to meet your partner's elbow in the ward off position. When your arms make the Ward Off position, step into the Bow Stance.

You should be able to recognise this movement from your Tai Chi form.

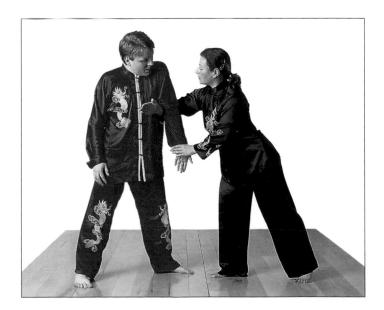

ROLL BACK

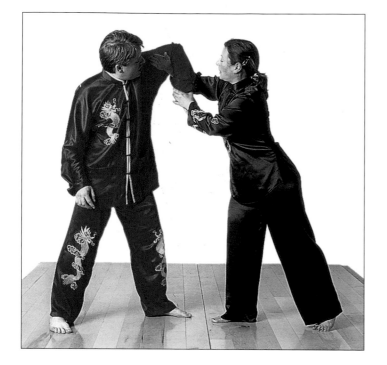

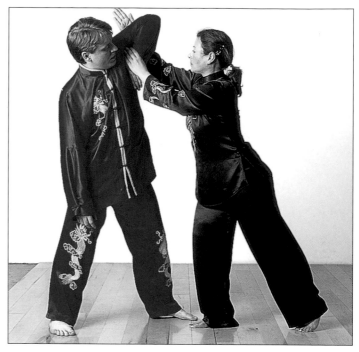

If you had just performed a successful Ward Off on an assailant, the combat sequence would be finished. For the purpose of understanding the applications of the moves, we will assume that you are unlucky enough to have an assailant who is a trained martial artist, and can escape from the elbow lock.

The way to escape from the elbow lock in the last move is to lift the elbow before the lock can be executed properly. In Tai Chi we never fight force with more force. Therefore, we will follow the elbow on its journey upwards. If you lift your left hand at the last part of the move, your partner's shoulder will rise. This will give the control of the situation back to you.

If your partner can extend fingers and push down, he may be able to escape. Again, the solution is to not use force. Just sink your weight back onto your left leg and move in to Roll Back. This will over-extend your partner's arm and lock it at the elbow.

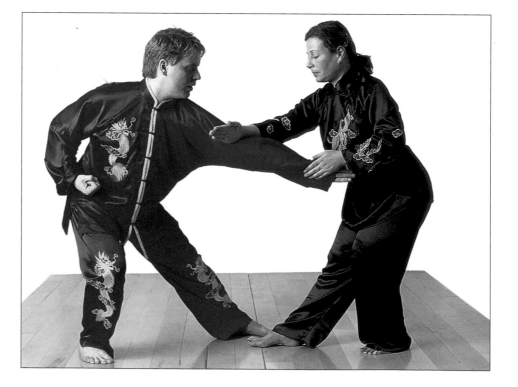

SQUEEZE

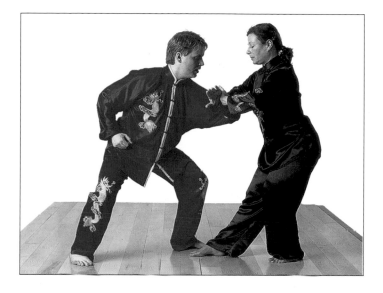

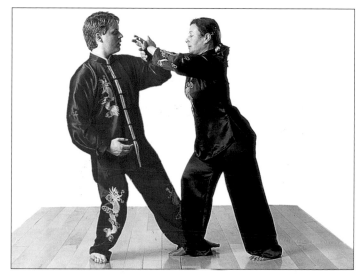

The only option that is open to your partner now is to try and unlock his elbow and push it into your abdomen. Neutralise this by dropping your right elbow.

When you drop your elbow and turn your waist, your left hand comes up to meet your right forearm. This puts you in position for a squeeze move. Push from the back leg to execute the squeeze.

PRESS

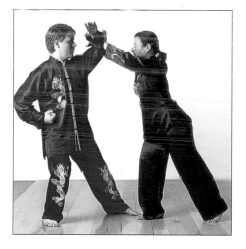

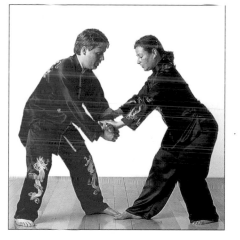

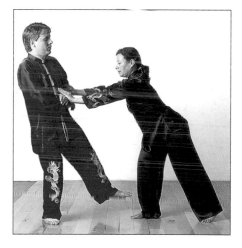

Your partner senses the squeeze approaching, so he deflects it with an upper block. This forces both of your hands to rise, so he tries a punch towards your stomach.

When you feel the squeeze movement rise, separate your hands. This will give you control over the forearm.

As the punch moves towards you, sink back and pull your arms on an inward arc. This will use your partner's arm to block his own punch. From the position where you are set back on your left leg, push forward into the Bow Stance. At the same time extend your arms to push. This double push will push your partner back to complete the sequence.

(9) SINGLE WHIP

Single Whip derives its name from the whip action of the arms if the move is performed at combat speed. This is another reminder to keep the arms soft. For a whip action to happen the whip must be flexible, otherwise it will have a much less powerful flick.

Single Whip is very useful as a standing exercise. If you can learn to stand in the *Single Whip* posture for any amount of time, your Bow Stance will improve. *Single Whip* will repeat again in the sequence. Points to Watch For, Visualisation and Applications are the same for both movements. A different application is shown on the second *Single Whip*.

THE MOVEMENT

During the movement of *Single Whip* you will perform another 180° turn like that in *Grasping the Sparrow's Tail*.

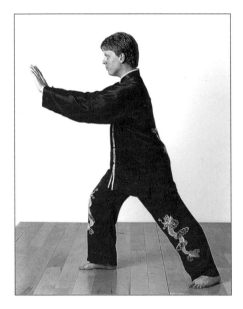

Start from the Push position at the end of the last move. Your right leg should be leading, and both of your arms extended.

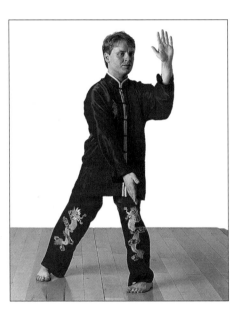

Turn your waist anti-clockwise and transfer your body weight onto your left leg. Keep your left arm high (to protect your face) and drop your right arm (to guard your groin) as you turn.

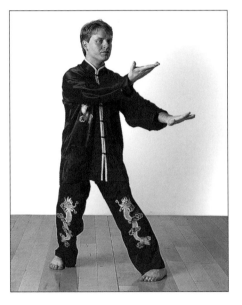

Turn your waist clockwise, and transfer the weight onto your right leg. Use this transfer of weight to push your left arm downwards and your right arm upwards.

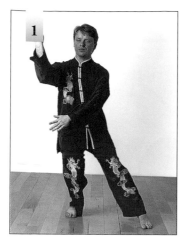
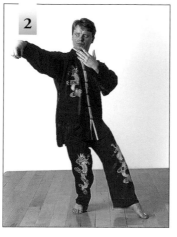
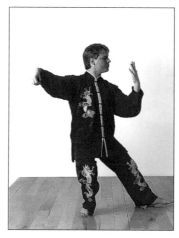
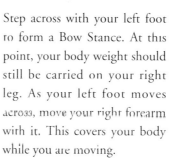

Form a hook with your right hand. Do this by touching all of your fingers onto your thumb and bending your wrist. (1) Point your right hand down and simultaneously lift your left heel. (2)

Step across with your left foot to form a Bow Stance. At this point, your body weight should still be carried on your right leg. As your left foot moves across, move your right forearm with it. This covers your body while you are moving.

Push your bodyweight from your right leg to your left leg to complete the Bow Stance. As your weight moves forward, extend your left hand in a spiral motion. Look in the direction of your left hand.

Visualisation

In the Ward Off posture, extend Energy through the fingers of your left hand. Imagine that the fingers of the ward-off arm are extending towards infinity.

Application

Your right hand can be used as strike, when in the hook position. This can only work if your wrist is completely bent over and your arm is relaxed. It should not be used to strike against anything that is hard.

POINTS TO WATCH OUT FOR:

- When stepping with your left leg, make sure that you step to the side as well as forward, otherwise your Bow Stance will finish too narrow.

- When making the hook with your right hand, keep your fingers straight. Do not lock your elbow, and keep your elbow pointing to the floor.

- Do not raise your left hand too high. The wrist should be slightly lower than shoulder height.

- Do not lean in to your left arm. Keep the posture square, with your waist pointing to the right.

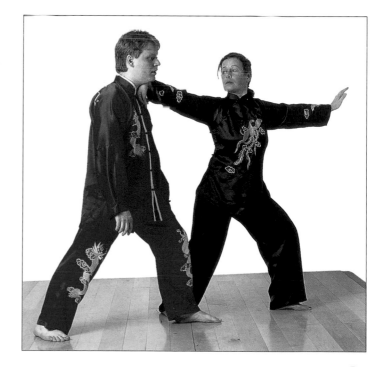

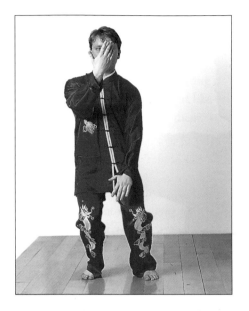

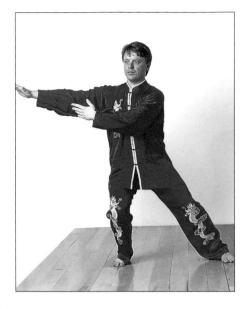

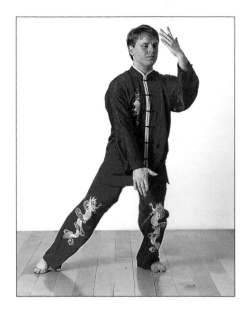

When you can rotate no farther in the anti-clockwise direction, change the rotation to clockwise. This will make your arms cross over and come back to the centre again. This time your right hand will guard your face and your left hand will guard your groin.

Continue rotating your waist clockwise. Again your arms will carry on past your centre as you turn. When you reach the point where you have to change the direction of rotation of your waist, extend your left leg sideways to step.

As you rotate your waist in the anti-clockwise direction, step in with your right leg to make the parallel stance. Your arms travel back to the centre in time with your waist.

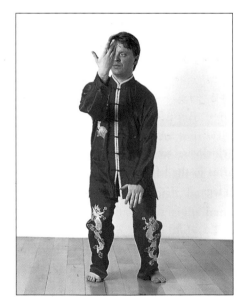

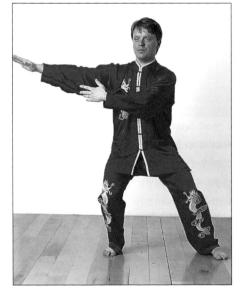

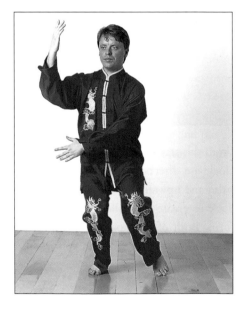

When you can rotate no farther in the anti-clockwise direction, change the rotation to clockwise. This will make your arms cross over and come back to the centre again. Again, your right hand will guard your face and your left hand will guard your groin.

Continue rotating your waist clockwise. Again the arms will carry on past your centre as you turn. When you reach the point where you have to change the direction of rotation of your waist, extend your left leg sideways to step.

As you rotate your waist in the anti-clockwise direction once more, step in with your right leg to make the parallel stance. Your arms travel back to the centre with your waist.

Visualisation

Feel the difference between Yin and Yang Energies with the arm movement. When your arms are at the side of your body, you should be on an outward breath. This is the Yang part of the movement. You should feel the arms extended. Remember that one of the attributes of Yang energy is expansion. Feel Energy expand through the arms as the breath travels outwards.

As you breathe in, imagine softness and contraction as the arms come back towards your centre. This part of the move should be the softest. Do not hold your arms out solidly in front of you.

With experience you will be able to feel Yin and Yang in all of the Tai Chi movements. *Waving Hands Like Clouds* is a good place to start the focus on these feelings, as the movement with the arms is relatively uncomplicated.

POINTS TO WATCH OUT FOR:

- Make the movement continuous. Your waist should keep moving and lead the movement of your arms. If you pause half way through the movement for equal weighting in your feet, the Energy will stop.

- When you move a foot, make sure that you are stable on your standing leg. If your weight is not carried fully on your standing leg you will lean or wobble.

- When you place your foot down, ensure that you follow the sequence of placing the toe first, then the heel and finally shift your weight.

- Keep your waist relaxed when performing the movement, otherwise your hips will poke out.

Application

If your opponent makes an attack to your chest with his or her right hand, the blow can be deflected and then re-directed with your right hand. This is an application of Ward Off, learned in *Grasping the Sparrow's Tail*.

The defence starts by intercepting the attack with your right hand. The turning of your waist will then divert the attack. When the attack has been diverted, your left arm will rise. This can be used as an attack to the elbow or to throw your opponent to one side. (1-3)

In this explanation, the opponent uses his or her right hand, and you deflect with your right hand. If you are attacked with the left hand, you can perform exactly the same technique with your left hand. The only difference is that you will need to turn your body the other way.

This technique is very versatile as a defence against many different sorts of attack. It will not work, however, unless you turn your waist with the movement. The most common mistake is to try and use the arms on their own, without letting the waist become involved. This will make the technique less effective, because you will not be able to stay soft.

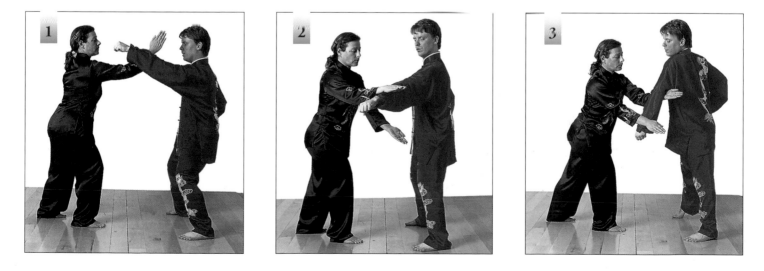

(11) SINGLE WHIP

This is a repeat movement. The movement is exactly the same as the one practised earlier. Notice how the movement of the *Single Whip* flows seamlessly with that of *Waving Hands like Clouds*.

THE MOVEMENT

Start from the third movement of *Waving Hands Like Clouds*. Your bodyweight is carried on your right leg. Your right hand is in the high position and your left hand is lower. Form a hook with your right hand. Do this by touching all of your fingers onto your thumb and bending your wrist. Point your right hand down and simultaneously lift your left heel. Step across with your left foot to form a Bow Stance. As yet, your bodyweight should still be carried on your right leg. As your left foot moves across, move your right forearm with it. This covers your body while you are moving. Push your bodyweight from your right leg to your left leg to complete the Bow Stance. As your weight moves forward, extend your left hand in a spiral motion. Look in the direction of your left hand. (1-6)

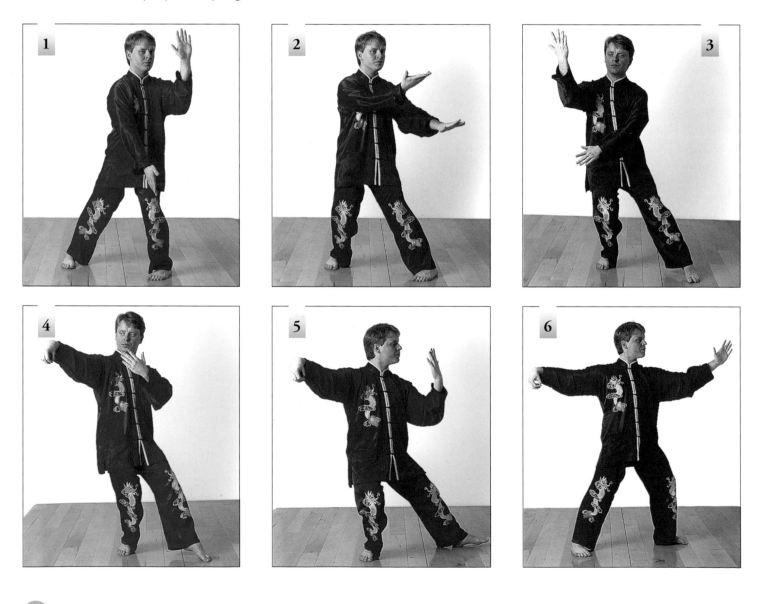

Visualisation

The *Single Whip* posture uses Energy travelling from both your left and the right hands. It is important that when you use the intent to move Energy through your hands you treat them both equally. To do this your body must be well centred and upright.

If you lean towards either hand, you will emphasise the energy in that hand. This will cause a depletion of Energy in the other.

Remain centred and calm when performing the move. This will help you to distribute Energy equally throughout your body.

POINTS TO WATCH OUT FOR:

- When stepping with your left leg, make sure that you step to the side as well as forward, otherwise your Bow Stance will finish too narrow.

- When making the hook with your right hand, keep your fingers straight. Do not lock your elbow, and keep it pointing to the floor.

- Do not raise your left hand too high. Your wrist should be slightly lower than shoulder height.

- Do not lean in to your left arm. Keep the posture square, with your waist pointing to the right.

Application

The left hand shows yet another application of Ward Off. If an opponent comes at you from the side, the fist is deflected with the Ward Off made with your left arm. This will throw the attacking arm to one side, which leaves your opponent vulnerable to your attack. This attack comes as a strike with the edge of your hand to the opponent's neck.

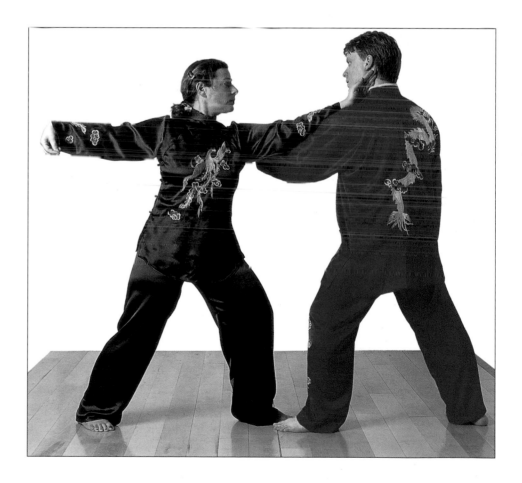

SECTION 3

The end of section 2 brings you to a point that is half way through the Simplified Tai Chi form. The sequence has by this time taught you all the basic techniques of Tai Chi. You will have also learned how to move forward, backward and sideways. After the first half of the Tai Chi form, there is much less repetition. A reason for this is that we are now simply re-applying what we already know to different parts of the form.

For example, there will shortly be two kicks to learn in the form. The kick is powered in exactly the same way as the Push technique that has already been featured within the form. The only difference is that the Push is being performed with your foot instead of your hand.

The same is also true of the stances. We will shortly be learning another stance — the Drop Stance. This is like a cross between the Bow Stance and the Empty Stance. Other than that, you already know all of the stances. The difference will be that you will learn how to use them in different ways.

At the moment, you may still feel that you are not sure whether your feet are in the correct position or not. This will start to become clearer as you work your way through the second half of the form.

(12) HIGH PAT ON HORSE

THE MOVEMENT

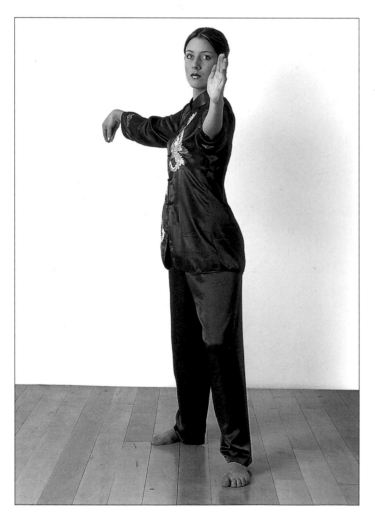

Start from the last movement, *Single Whip*.

Shift all of your body weight on to your left leg. Do this by moving your waist forward and keeping your torso in an upright position. As you move forward, rotate your fore arms so that the palms of your hands face upwards. As your weight moves forward on to your left leg, move your right leg half of a step closer to the left. Touch the floor with the ball of your right foot, but do not rest any of your weight to it yet.

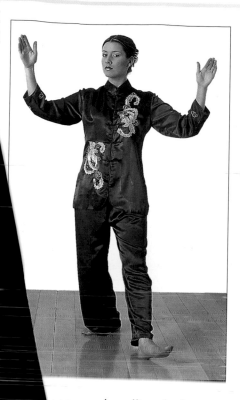

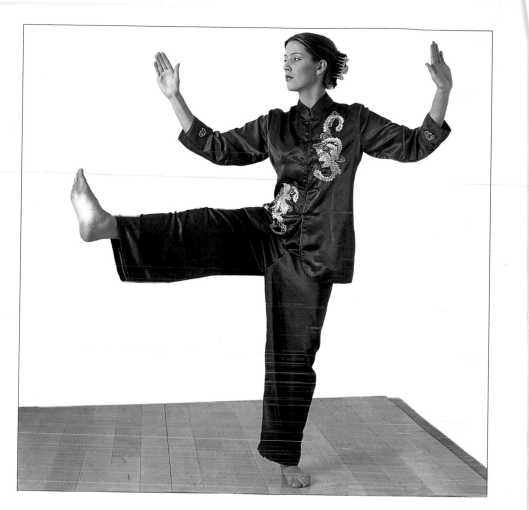

...e arms up by rolling the forearms
...ds. As your forearms move
..., sink your body weight on to
... leg, so that it carries most of
... weight.

Straighten your left leg to lift your body upwards. Lift the knee of your right leg and kick to a 45° angle with your right heel.

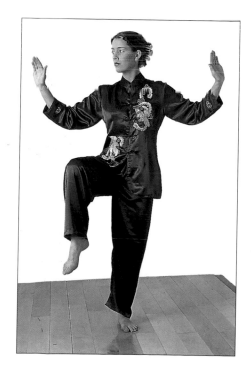

When you have done the kick, bend your right leg again. Do not leave your right leg in the extended position once you have done the kick. As your leg kicks out, sink your shoulders.

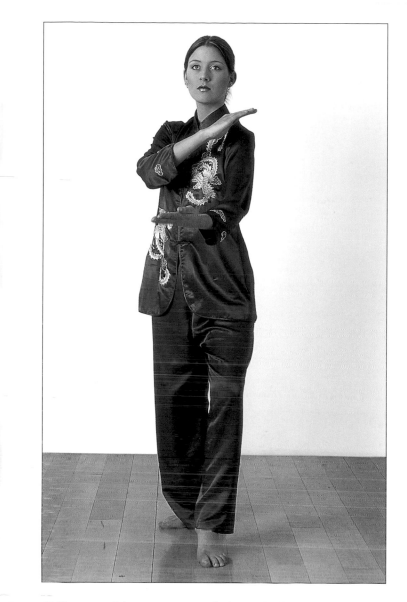

Shift your weight on to your right leg and adjust your left leg so that you are in Empty Stance. The ball of your left foot should be touching the floor and the heel slightly raised. There should be no weight carried on your left leg. As you move in to the Empty Stance, bend your right arm so the palm of your hand is facing downwards and is in front of your chest. Your torso should face approximately 45° to the right.

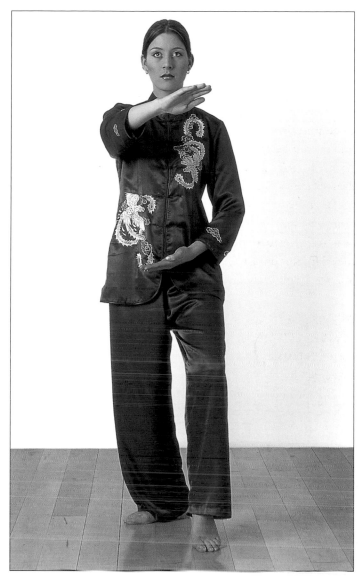

Turn your torso to face the front. As you do this, sink your body onto your right leg. This causes your body to move in a downward spiral that provides the power for your arm movement. Your arms will move at the same time as your body moves down in a spiral. Both of your arms need to move in a circle. The right arm moves in a circle away from your body and the left arm moves in a circle towards your waistline. Finish with your right arm extended and your left arm drawn in to your body. Stand in the Empty Stance.

Visualisation

When you perform *High Pat on Horse*, both of your arms and your Tan Tien will be moving in a spiral at the same time.

When you are first learning the movement, feel a connection between your arms. Feel them move together and not as separate units moving independently of each other.

When you have become familiar with the feeling of your arms working together on this movement, extend the idea to your Tan Tien. The movement of the arms should be in co-ordination with the movement of your Tan Tien. If you can feel they are all working together as a part of the same thing, you will have started to move from the Tan Tien, rather than simply waving your arms. When you are in your final position, extend Chi through your fingertips on the right hand.

Application

If your left hand has been grabbed from the Single Whip posture, the first thing that you should do is to turn your forearm over. This will have the effect of weakening your opponent's grip on you. As you turn the arm, step forward and prepare to strike with your right hand. When you sink your body in to the empty stance, withdraw your left arm by pulling your elbow in to your body. This will have the effect of pulling your opponent down so that you can strike to the neck. (1-3)

POINTS TO WATCH OUT FOR:

- Keep your back straight and your head up during the movement and in the final posture.

- Move from the waist. This will help you keep upright and to co-ordinate your movements.

- In the final part of the movement, do not straighten your right arm. The right arm should be extended, but never straight in any Tai Chi movements.

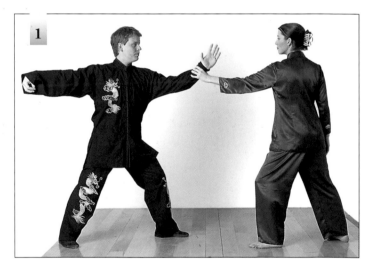

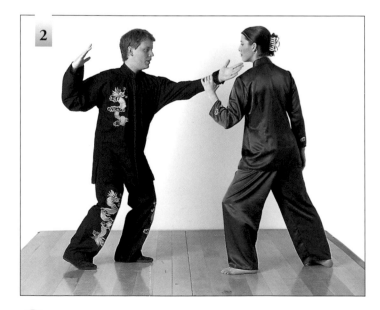

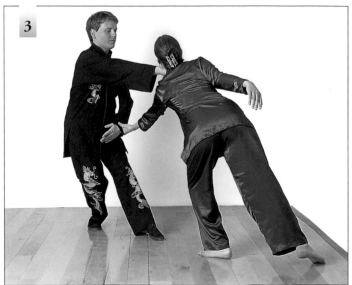

(13) KICK WITH THE RIGHT HEEL

THE MOVEMENT

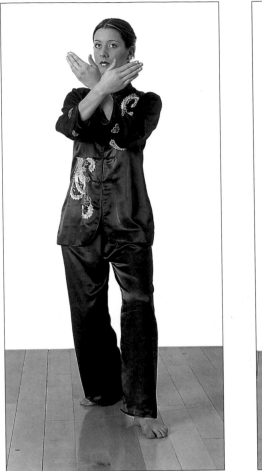

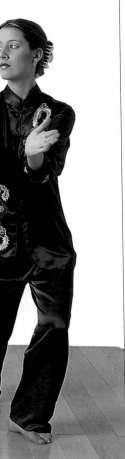

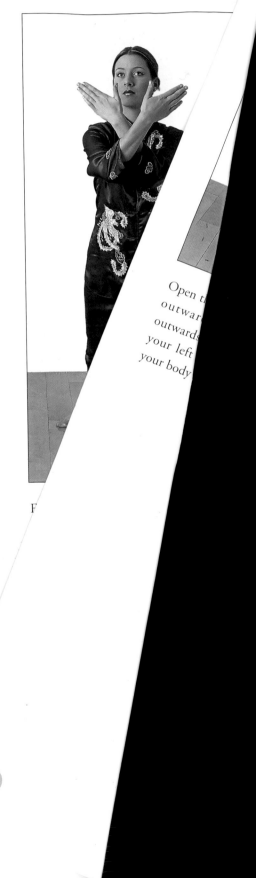

Start from *High Pat on Horse*. Sink your torso down slightly. As your torso sinks, turn your right forearm so that your right palm faces you. Lift your left forearm so that it crosses your right forearm. The left forearm should be on the outside.

Step forward with your left leg into the Bow Stance. As you step forward sweep your arms forward at the side of your body.

Open t
outwar
outwards
your left
your body

Visualisation

The most difficult aspect of this kick is keeping straight when you are kicking and timing.

When you kick out with the heel you need to keep your body straight. If you do not, the balance will be affected adversely. This can deceive you into thinking that you can kick high when you cannot. As you kick out, feel the weight of your body push through your heel. If you can feel your body weight push through your heel, it means that your body is in alignment. If you cannot feel this you may be leaning forwards or backwards. When you can feel the weight working through the heel, imagine that your Energy extends from your heel into the floor. This will increase your feeling of Rooting.

The timing of the kick should mean that it comes after the arms have opened. Imagine that your arms are opening a pathway for your leg to follow. If the pathway is blocked, then you cannot perform the kick.

POINTS TO WATCH OUT FOR:

- As mentioned earlier, a common mistake is to lean the body when you kick. Avoid this by not trying to kick high. As your muscles become trained, the kick will get higher. It is better to perform a low kick and be correct than to try higher kicks that are wrong.

- In the final kick position, both legs are the same. They should be straight but not locked.

- Do not move your right arm out at the same time as the kick. The sequence is to move the arms and then perform the kick.

- In the final position your right arm should be slightly to the right hand side of your kicking leg. It is important to not open up your arms too far. Remember the third Essence.

- Try to co-ordinate all of the movement from your waist.

Application

If you are attacked from the right-hand side with a fist, the first action is to block the fist with your right forearm. The action of the block should roll with the Energy of your opponent's fist, so that they become over-extended. This will open a highly vulnerable target area for a kick. (1-2)

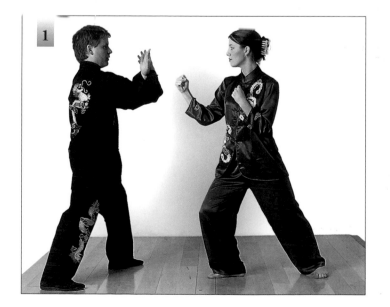
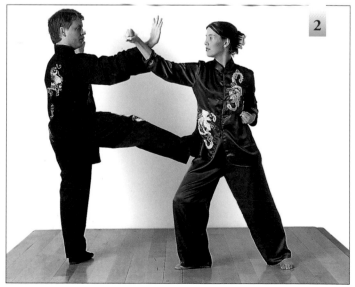

(14) STRIKE OPPONENT'S EARS WITH BOTH FISTS

THE MOVEMENT

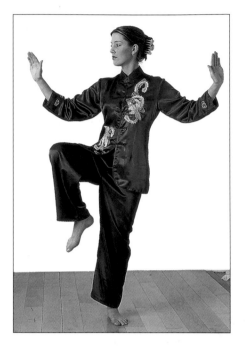

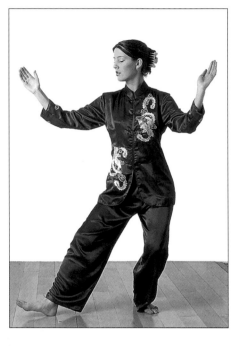

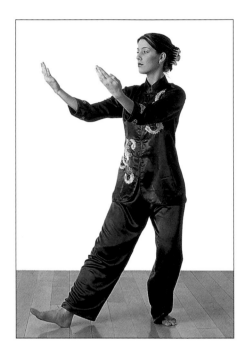

Start from the previous posture, *Kick with Right Heel.* You have just performed the kick and withdrawn it. Your knee is high and your arms are extended.

Bend your left leg so that your torso sinks downwards. As your torso sinks, extend your right heel forward and slightly to the right.

Simultaneous with the extension of your right heel, move both of your arms so that they are extended in front of you with the palms facing upwards.

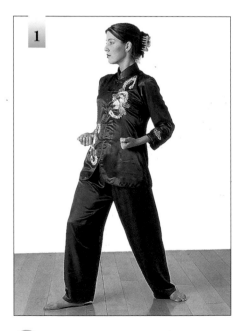

Lower the toes of your right foot, so that it is flat on the floor. As your toes move to the floor, clench your fists but keep them relaxed. Draw your elbows back to your body to prepare for the punch. Your forearms should be facing upward.(1)

When the forearms are fully withdrawn, turn them so that they face the floor. This is the moment that you push all your weight from your left leg to your right, to drive the double punch forward. The punch should finish around eye level, with approximately the distance of two fists between your hands. (2)

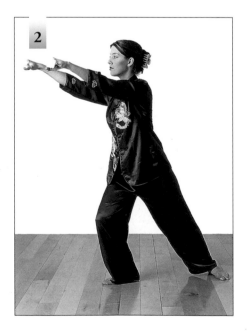

Visualisation

When your fists move forward, they should move in an arc. This arc, however, should be quite shallow. It is not correct to move the arms in a large circle, as this would be too easy for an opponent to stop.

It is tempting to make your fists too tight. This is especially true if you have studied a 'hard' martial art such as Karate. The punch Tai Chi works in a different way to a 'hard' punch. A way to keep the punch soft is to not focus your attention on your fists alone. Imagine that you are creating a surge of Energy from your Tan Tien that is moving out through the fist.

Application

The application for this posture is as simple as its name suggests. You will punch your opponent's ears with both fists. Keep the arc of travel towards the ears shallow so that it is more difficult to block. (1-3)

It is important to maintain the arc, as this will allow the punch to be used as a block when you become more advanced.

POINTS TO WATCH OUT FOR:

- Keep your shoulders down. When the punch rises to the high position, you still need to keep your shoulders low. If this feels difficult, do not punch as high. Go to your own limit. It is better to be aware of the fact that your shoulders need to loosen, than it is to deceive yourself by raising them.

- Co-ordinate the movement of your legs with the movement of your arms. Do not allow the punch to 'overtake' the movement of your legs.

- In the final position, you should be facing an angle of 45° from the direction of your movement.

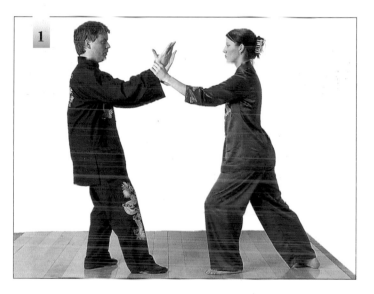

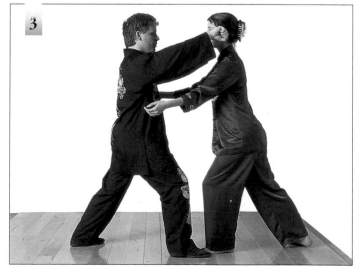

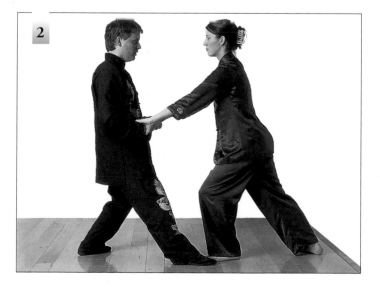

(15) KICK WITH LEFT HEEL

THE MOVEMENT

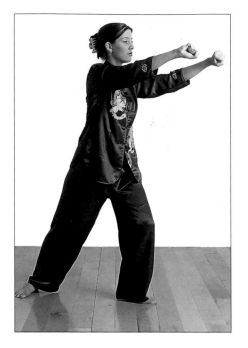 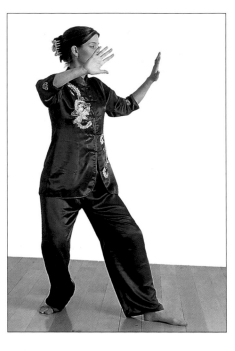 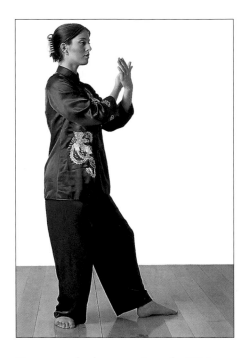

This second kick starts from the double punch position of the previous posture.

Relax and sink your waist slightly. Open your hands as you sink.

Turn your body approximately 90° in an anti-clockwise direction. The movement of your waist transfers your weight on to your left leg. As your body turns, move your forearms in a large arc that finishes in front of your body, at the end of the turn. Your left forearm should be in front of your right forearm and they should both be at chest height. Your body should face an angle of 45° to the left.

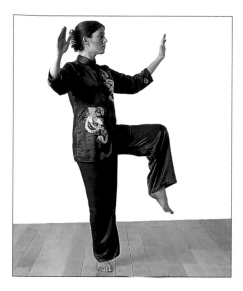

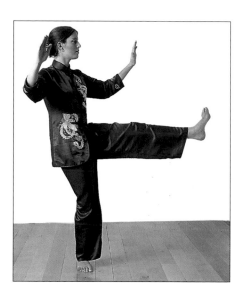

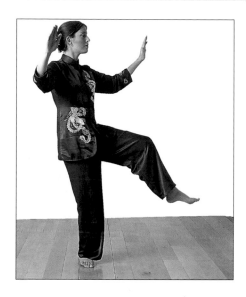

Turn your body so that your body weight transfers back to your right leg. As your weight shifts, lift up your left heel and open your arms.

Lift up your knee and kick with your left heel. The kick should be at an angle of 90° to the left. As you kick out with your heel, sink your shoulders.

Withdraw the kick by bending your left knee.

Visualisation

The visualisation for the left heel kick is exactly the same as for the right heel kick.

Most people find that it is easier to kick with one leg than the other. Even after years of practice it is common to have a favourite leg for kicking. Whilst this is an acceptable fact, it is also one that you can use to your advantage.

If you have a favourite leg, then it is quite tempting to train only with that leg because it feels easier and with little effort soon starts to look good. This has obvious disadvantages.

A better approach is to train with your weaker leg more, to get the kick correct for that leg. You will find that this will teach you more about your body and the leg that did not receive quite as much attention will have improved without you having to try very hard.

Application

Applications of the left and right kicks are exactly the same.

POINTS TO WATCH OUT FOR:

• The mechanics and Energy movements for each of the kicks are exactly the same.

• Now that you have become more accustomed to the idea of kicking, try and work out the reasoning behind these points. Use the Ten Essences as a guideline. You will probably find you need to remind yourself of other issues.

• These will be YOUR lessons from the kick. If you can work out your specific faults and requirements, you will be learning how to teach yourself.

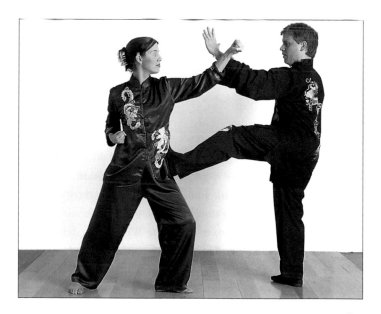

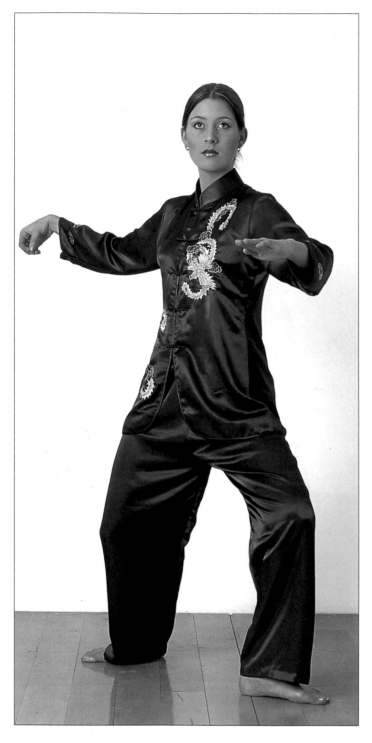

Visualisation

When you are sinking your weight into the low position, you are storing up Energy in your right leg. This works in the same way as when a spring is compressed.

If a spring is compressed, it will try to convert stored-up potential energy into kinetic energy by expanding. This is how the fingertips of your left hand are thrust forward using Energy that was stored when you sank into the Drop Stance.

Imagine that it is not simply the storage of potential energy and the release of kinetic energy that is taking place. When you sink, you are compressing your body. This compression of Energy is the Yin part of an Energy exchange. It is preparing for the expansive Yang part of the Energy exchange, where your fingers thrust forward. Viewed in this way, you are attuning yourself to the primal forces of the Universe — Yin and Yang.

Points to Watch Out For:

- The most important thing to be careful of when performing *Snake Creeps Down* is not to sink too low. If you go too low, then it will be impossible for you to keep your torso straight during the movement. The movement will become weaker and you lose the intent of the movement. Keep your head up and your spirit high.

- When you thrust the fingers of your left hand forward, the elbow should be in line with your fingertips. This will make the thrust stronger and follows the principle of Push Energy.

- When you squat down, your rear right foot should be turned outwards, otherwise you will not be able to bend your right leg and squat down.

- In the final position, most of your body weight should be on your left or leading leg.

Push your body weight forward from your right leg to your left leg. This will thrust the fingers of your left hand forward for a strike. The right arm is still not required to make any adjustments. Adjust your right foot to a 45° angle on the final part of the movement. Do this by pushing your toes forward. Do not make the adjustment by sliding your heel back, as this neutralises the Energy that you are moving forward.

Application

If your left hand is grabbed, you can escape or take your opponent off-balance by sinking into the Drop Stance. This will put you in the position of being able to thrust the fingers of your left hand forward into the groin or abdomen area. If the movement is completed with your full body weight behind it, your partner will be 'pacified'. (1-3)

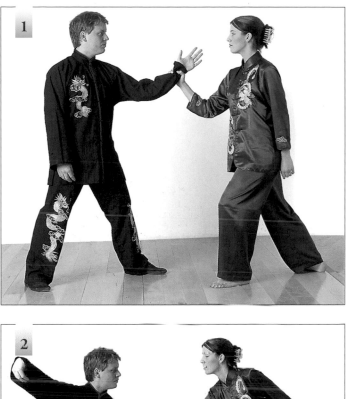

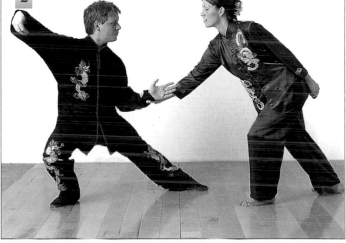

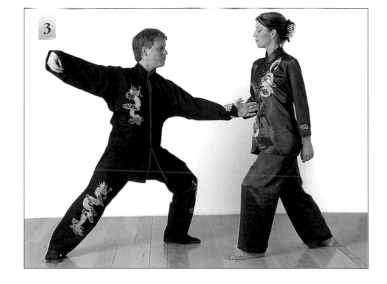

(17) GOLDEN ROOSTER STANDS ON ONE LEG (RIGHT SIDE)

THE MOVEMENT

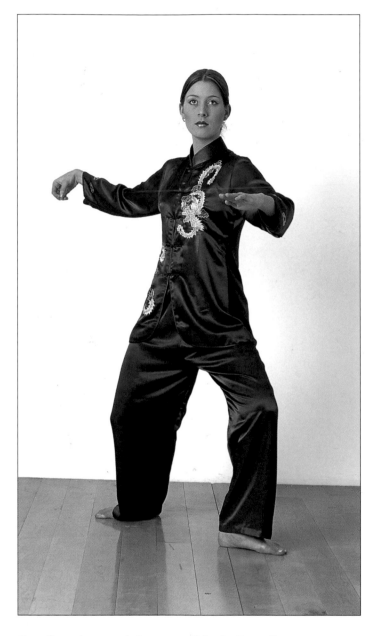 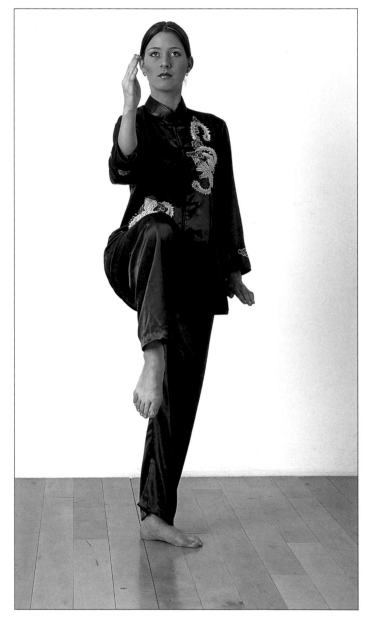

Start from the extended posture of *Snake Creeps Down.*

Keep your body weight forward on your left leg. Push your heel onto the floor and open your toes by turning them to the left at an angle of 45°. Release the hook made by your right hand. Press downward with your left heel and move your waist forward.

This will enable you to lift your body up on to your left leg. your right knee should be forward and lifted quite high. The fingertips of your right hand should be extended forward with your elbow pointing downwards. Press down with your right hand.

Visualisation

Balance can sometimes be difficult when learning this posture. Imagine that your left hand is being used to lean on something solid, to help to keep you steady.

This has the effect of helping you to ground your Energy better, so that your balance improves.

POINTS TO WATCH OUT FOR:

- Keep your head upright and your eyes steady. If you do not keep your torso straight and your spirit high, balancing will be difficult.

- The right knee is raised, but not to a position that makes your torso lean backwards. If you find that your torso is leaning when you lift your right knee, practice with it lower. After a while your muscles will grow accustomed to the movement, and your balance will improve. This will allow you to lift your knee higher.

- The movement of this posture involves a transition from a low posture to a high posture. This can create difficulties with co-ordination. Keep the movement coming from your waist to help keep the movement smooth.

- If your mind is not balanced, then your body will be difficult to balance. If you find that your mind is full of other things whilst practising your Tai Chi, it will make balancing more difficult. Take a deep breath, relax your mind and try again. Remember that it can take time for you to be able to let go of your internal dialogue, so do not try to rush.

Application

The opening part of the movement with your left hand is used as a block to your opponent's attack. You can then respond by lifting up your leg to strike their side with your knee, or into the groin with your foot. (1-2) Alternatively a hand strike to the throat is effective. (3)

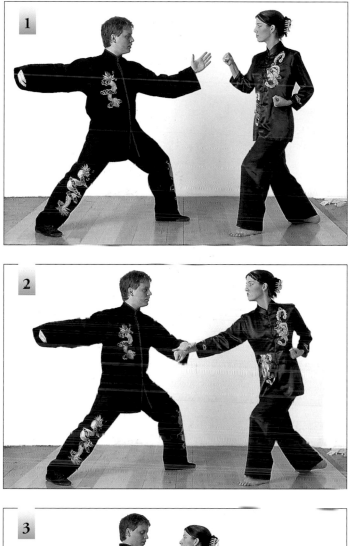

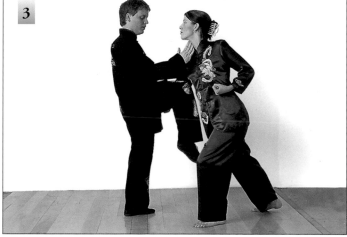

(18) SNAKE CREEPS DOWN (RIGHT SIDE)

THE MOVEMENT

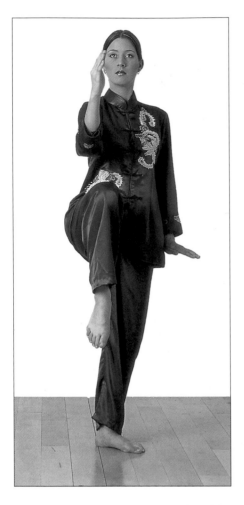 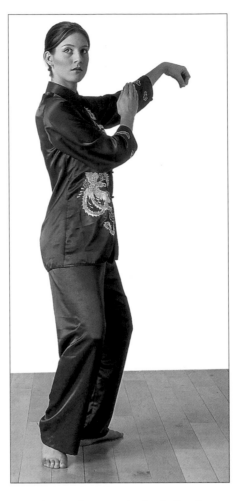 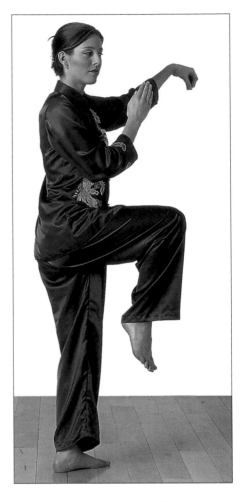

Start from the final position of *Golden Rooster Stands on One Leg*.

Touch the floor with the ball of your right foot. Do not place any weight on it yet. Lift up on to the balls of both of your feet and turn your body 135° in an anti-clockwise direction. As your body turns, make a hook with your left hand and extend it forward. Your right arm bends at the elbow, so that your fingers point upwards.

As you lower your left heel, lift your right knee. You should now be in the same position as at the start of *Snake Creeps Down* on the left side except that you are standing on your left leg instead of your right leg.

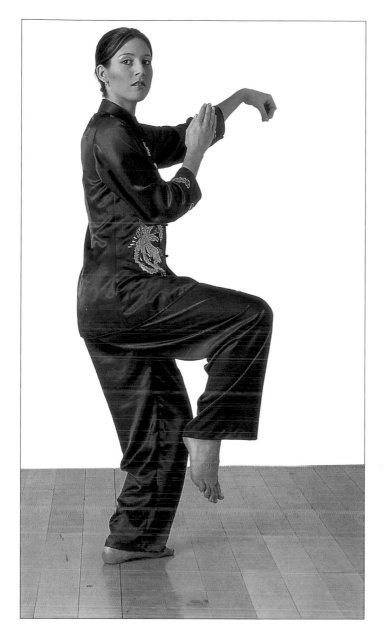

When you have aligned your body to the 45° angle, sink down on your left leg. As your torso sinks, extend your right leg out in a straight line. Touch the ball of your right foot on to the floor. The toes of your right foot should be in line with the heel of your left. After the ball of your right foot has made contact with the floor, keep sinking your weight. This will push the heel of the right foot, putting it on the same angle as the left. In this transitional part of the movement, your feet are parallel with each other. Turn your waist clockwise, so that your body faces to the right. Simultaneous with the movement of your waist, pick up your right toes and turn them to face the right.

The movement of the right arm takes its timing from the waist. As your waist turns bring your fingers in a downward arc that finishes pointing in the same direction as your body. The arm should be positioned just inside the right leg. Your body weight should still be firmly held on the left leg. Keep your back straight and do not lean. Push your body weight forward from your left leg to your right leg. This will thrust the fingers of your right hand forward for a strike. The left arm is still not required to make any adjustments. Adjust your left foot to a 45° angle on the final part of the movement. Do this by pushing the toes forward.

Note that all visualisations, points to watch for and applications are exactly the same on the left side as the right side. Please refer to *Snake Creeps Down* on the Left Side if you require revision of these items.

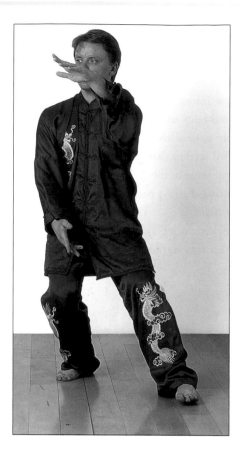

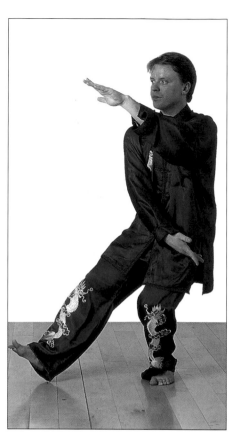

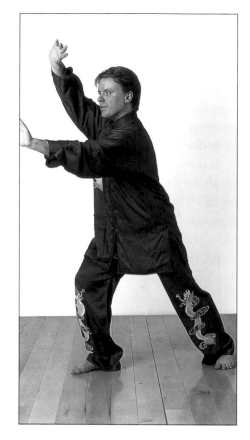

Sink your body weight on your right leg. As your weight sinks, extend your left heel forward and to the side. Round your arms, leaving your left arm higher than your right.

Lower the toes of your left foot, so that it is flat on the floor. Move all of your body weight on to your left leg and step out to 45° angle with your right leg. This is to prepare for a Bow Stance that faces to 45° angle on the right side. Be careful to place the right foot in the correct position.

Push from your right heel to move your torso forward. As your waist moves forward your right arm rises above your head and then your left hand pushes forward. This is the completion of the first stance. You should be in Bow Stance, facing a 45° angle, have your right arm above your head and push with your left palm.

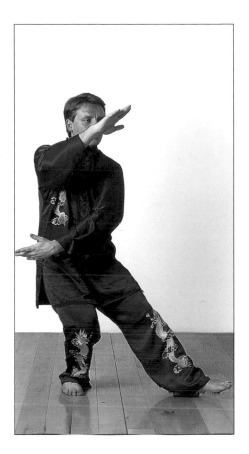

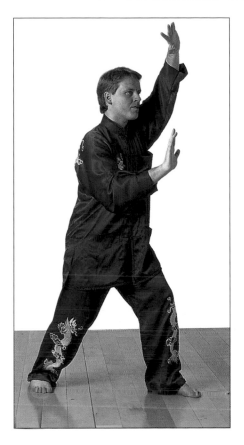

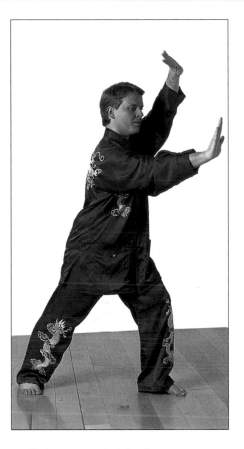

Move your weight back onto your left leg. As you move backwards let your arms become more rounded and lift your right toes. Lower the toes of your right foot, so that it is flat on the floor. When your foot is flat, turn your waist in an anti-clockwise direction. This will transfer your weight on to your right leg.

When your body weight is carried on your right leg, step out with your left for a 45° Bow Stance to the left.

Push from your left heel to move your torso forward. As your waist moves forward your left arm rises above your head and then your right hand pushes forward. This is the completion of the second and final stance of the movement. You should be in Bow Stance, facing a 45° angle, have your left arm above your head and push with your right palm.

Visualisation

Project Energy from the hand that is performing the push. Imagine that your hand extends further than flesh and bone. Feel Energy moving through your arm and coming out through the centre of your palm.

Feel that your legs support the hand in the high position. If the Energy is continuous through your body, it should feel strong without the need for force.

Application

If an attempt were made to strike your face, you could deflect the movement by using the high Ward Off, used in the sequence. This would then leave you with the opportunity to strike the chest with the palm of your hand. (1-2)

POINTS TO WATCH OUT FOR:

- The fact that *Fair Lady Works the Shuttles* is working on 45° angles frequently causes confusion. It is normal that people no longer stand in a correct Bow Stance when this movement is being learned. If you find that you make this error, then try to pay attention to where you place your stepping leg.

- Keep your shoulders down. It is common for beginners to raise the shoulder of the blocking arm. Be on your guard against this.

- The blocking arm uses Ward Off Energy and the palm uses Pressing Energy. Try to feel the similarities between this movement and others that use the same Energies.

- The higher Ward Off arm needs to block before the palm can strike. Try to incorporate this into your timing of the movement.

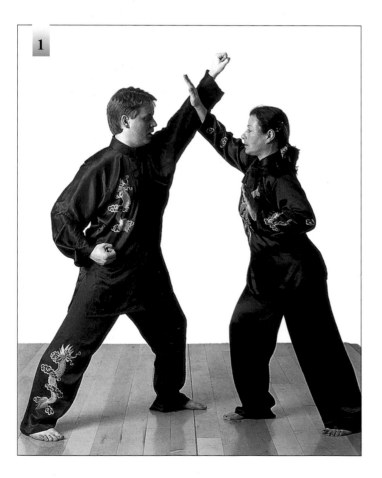

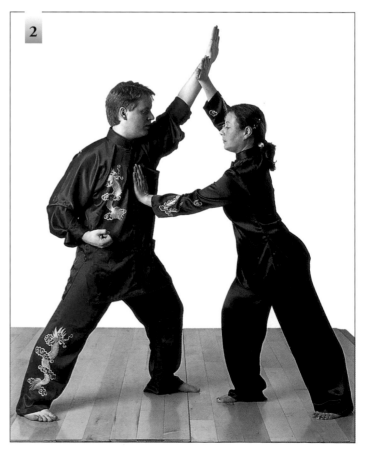

(21) NEEDLE AT THE BOTTOM OF THE SEA

The Needle, in this allegory is that of the tapestry artist, and represents original thought. Everybody is capable of producing original thought that can be transformed into a work of art. The 'Art' may be as simple as the way that you live your life.

To produce a work of art, one requires inspiration. To gain inspiration you must reach into the subconscious, represented by the Sea in this allegory. *The Needle at the Sea Bottom* can therefore be interpreted as reaching into your subconscious to retrieve original thought or ideas.

THE MOVEMENT

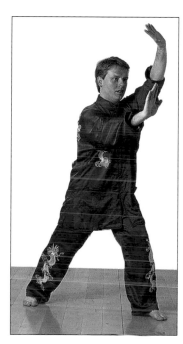

Start from the final position of *Fair Lady Works Shuttles*, where your right palm is extended and your left forearm is in the 'high' position.

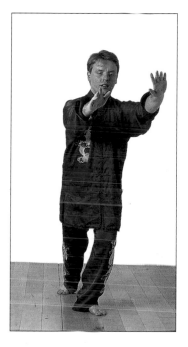

Push all of your weight onto your left leg. Turn your waist in a clockwise direction. Move your right foot to a position that is approximately in line with your left heel. Touch the floor with the ball of your right foot. Relax your elbows, so that when your weight shifts, your arms move with them. Your arms finish in a position where both are level, and extended in front of your chest.

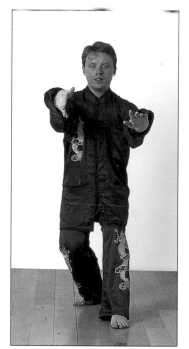

Shift your weight back onto your right leg. This should put you into the well-practised Empty Stance. Withdraw both of your elbows slightly. Keep the palm of your left hand facing the floor. Turn the palm of your right hand to your left. This will cause your wrist to bend when you sink your elbow.

Sink down on your right leg, and bend your waist. Your waist should work like a hinge on a door. You need to bend from your waist, but keep your back straight. Point the fingers of your right hand to the floor. The left palm stays flat.

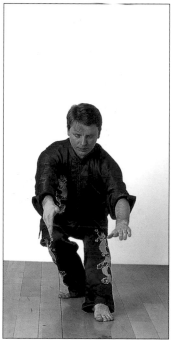

Visualisation

Feel your Tan Tien sink. This will help you to co-ordinate the movement from your waist.

As you sink, there is a temptation to lose the first Essence—*Lift the Head to Raise the Spirit*. Prevent this from happening by raising the spirit before you start the movement. This internal movement of the Spirit will be reflected when you perform the movement by your external frame.

POINTS TO WATCH OUT FOR:

- A common mistake with this movement is to arch the back. This gives the appearance that you have sunk lower. The truth is that your posture has become weaker and you are off-balance. Avoid this situation by observing the First Essence and keeping your back straight.

- When you sink at the end of the movement, all your weight should be carried on your right leg. This will make your right thigh muscle work harder than at any other point in the form. When you start to learn the movement, do not sink too low. This will allow you greater control over the movement. Your range of movement will increase gradually as your legs get stronger.

- When you move your right arm, it should travel in an arc. Do not over-emphasise the arc, otherwise your shoulders may be forced to rise.

- Your left arm follows the movement of your right arm. The size of the movement is smaller. Do not forget your left arm and let it become static.

Application

If your opponent grabs your right hand, you can instantly weaken their grip by pointing your fingers to the floor. If you follow this by sinking your body, it will pull your partner down and control their arm. Further control can be exercised on your partner by placing your left palm on the inside of their elbow. (1-3)

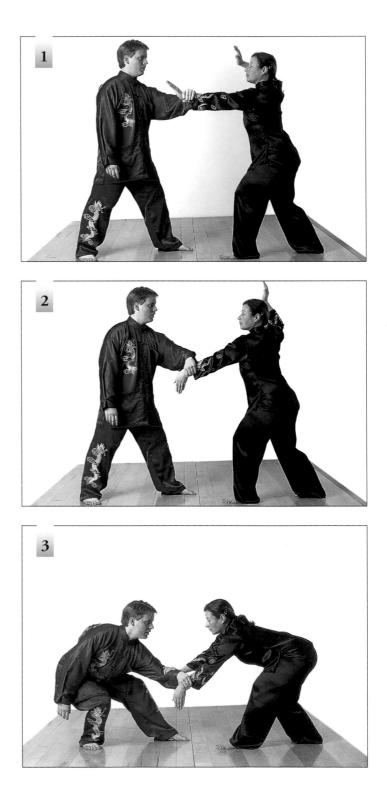

(22) Fan Through the Back

When you have reached for your *Needle at the Sea Bottom*, and received your inspiration, it needs to be expressed. This can provide inspiration to others and yourself to try and attain new levels of skill.

A common Chinese Art form is fan painting. The allegory for this movement is that the fan painting has been completed when the artist has received the required inspiration.

The image of immersing oneself into the subconscious and displaying the results was thematic in the sequence *Snake Creeps Down*, followed *by Golden Rooster Stands on One Leg.*

The Movement

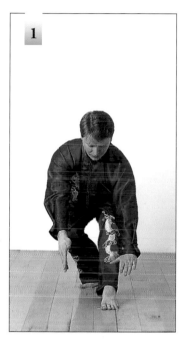

Start from the low position of *Needle at the Sea Bottom.*

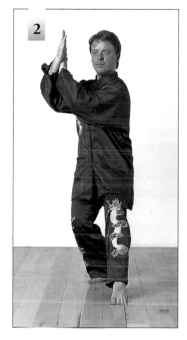

Push down on your right leg to straighten your torso. Ensure that the movement is generated from your legs and waist. As your torso lifts, raise your right arm to the side of your body. Place your left palm near to the wrist on your inner right forearm.

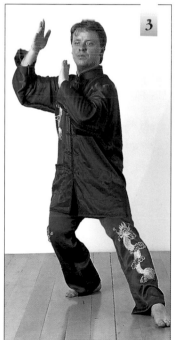

Step with your left leg, to prepare for the Bow Stance. Move your right forearm so that the palm faces outwards. Move your left hand to a position that is just inside the left shoulder.

Push your body weight from your right leg to your left leg. This will make your waist turn in a clockwise direction. Push the edge of your left hand forward and pull your right palm back to a position near your ear. Look in the direction of your left hand. Your waist should face your right.

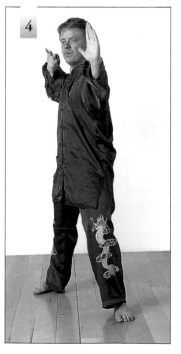

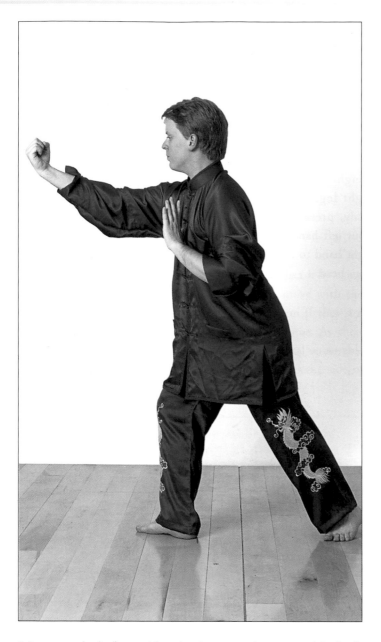

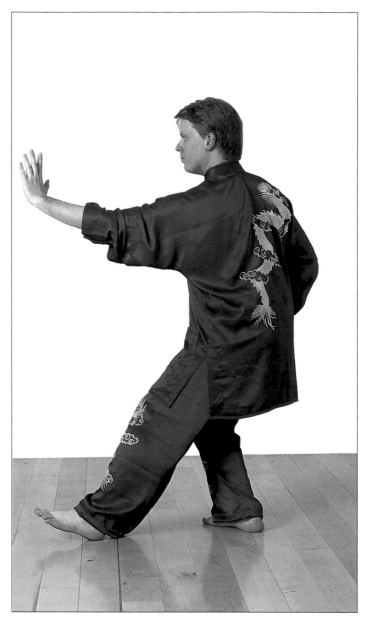

Move your body forward by pivoting around on your right heel. As your body turns, allow it to turn your foot to a 45° angle. The turning of your body will transfer your body weight on to your right leg. Use this momentum to drive your right fist forward in an arc. The arc of the movement follows a line through the middle of your chest.

Allow your left palm to sink to a position that is near to the body and just below your shoulder. Step forward with your left leg and simultaneously push your left hand forward. Your left foot moves to a position that is ready to be pushed forward into the Bow Stance. The toes of your left foot are raised. As your left hand moves forward, pull your right elbow back to your body. This is the preparation for the punch. The correct position for your fist is with the knuckles vertical and your thumb higher than your little finger.

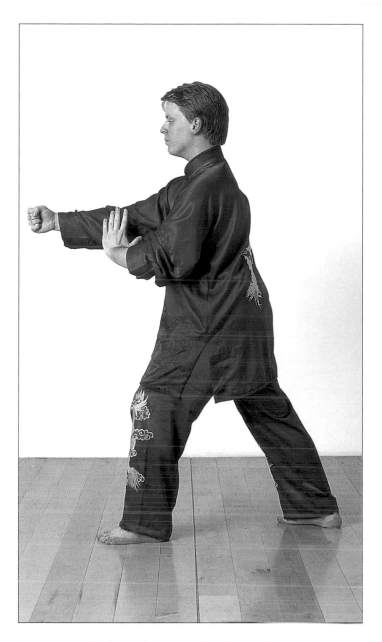

Push your body forward into the Bow Stance. Your body weight should become mostly balanced on your left leg. Use this forward shift of your body weight to drive the punch forward with your right hand. As the right-hand punch moves forward, bend your left elbow. This moves your left palm into a position that is close to your right forearm.

Visualisation

When you make the final punch for this pattern of movements, the fist and elbow travel outwards in a straight line. The movement of the fist is identical to a battering ram.

This may cause confusion at first, because Tai Chi movement is generally in circles and arcs. Straight lines are usually a sign that something is incorrect. If you think about the source of the movement, you will see that the straight-line part of the movement is a result of many different curves added together.

A good analogy to help understand the movement is to think about a car engine. The circular motion of a car's wheel derives from the linear motion of the engine cylinder. The cylinder in the engine of a car moves up and down. It is connected through various couplings and gears to the drive shaft. The drive shaft will then transfer rotational energy to the wheels.

The Tai Chi punch is the same, but in reverse. The original source of Energy is the Tan Tien, which is rotating. This rotational Energy is transmitted through your body, shoulder and upper arm. This will then drive your fist and elbow forward like the car's piston or cylinder.

POINTS TO WATCH OUT FOR:

- When your turn your body on the first part of the movement, look forward. Do not look down at your right hand.

- Keep your body straight when transferring your weight.

- When you push your left hand forward, your left leg should move simultaneously. If they do not move together, the top and bottom halves of your body are not co-ordinated.

- On the final punch, do not lock your elbow or push your shoulder forward.

Application

If your opponent attacks with their right hand, deflect it by using Squeeze Energy. Your right hand continues to move with the direction of their attack. (1-2) Do not try to pull them if they are already coming to you, otherwise you will use force. As their attack is drawn in and re-directed, (3) it will leave several vulnerable strike points open. The left palm can then strike to the side of your opponent's body. (4-5)

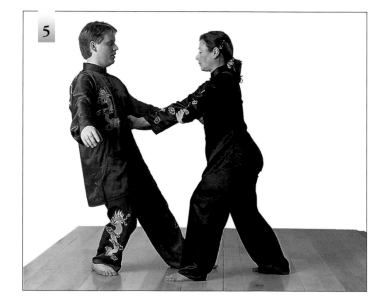

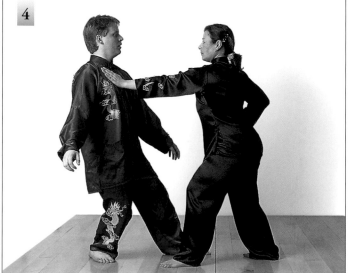

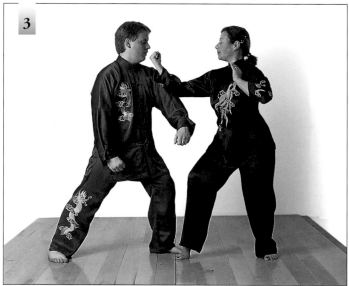

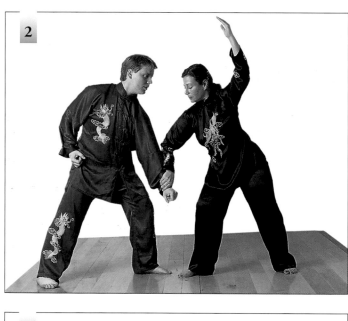

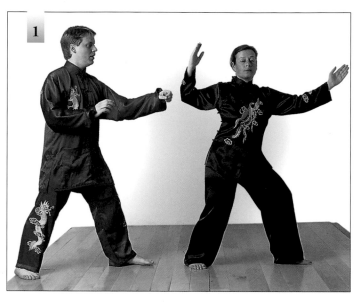

(24) APPARENT CLOSE-UP

THE MOVEMENT

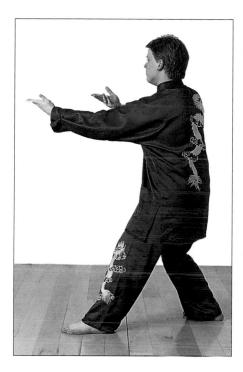

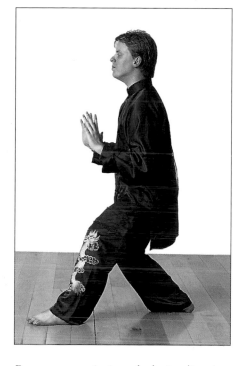

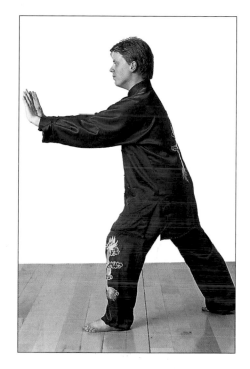

Start from the final punch of the previous movement. Turn both of your forearms over so that both palms face upwards.

Rotate your waist in a clockwise direction so that your left hand moves forward and your right hand moves back to a position near your left elbow. Sink your weight slightly on your right leg. This turns your waist in an anti-clockwise direction. Bring your palms parallel, ready for a double push.

Push from your right heel. Force your body weight on to your left leg to perform the double push. This part of the movement is exactly the same as the double push at the end of *Grasping the Sparrows Tail.*

Visualisation

When you withdraw your arms, make sure that you have intent in both of the arms. It is easy to make the mistake of letting one arm lead the other.

This is made easy by imagining that both forearms are travelling in their own circles. If you feel that there is circular movement within both of your arms, they will be used correctly.

POINTS TO WATCH OUT FOR:

- When you withdraw your arms, do not bring your right arm too close to the body. You should be able to maintain an underarm gap at all times.

- When you push, move from the waist to ensure that your torso is co-ordinated with your legs.

Application

If you were to attempt the punch from the previous sequence, there is always a chance that it will not hit the target. If your fist is straight out in front of you, it is easy for your opponent to grab your wrist.

Rotating your forearms would immediately weaken the grab. The movement of your left hand can then be used to brush your opponent's hand away. This is followed by a push to make sure that you can get them away from you. (1-3)

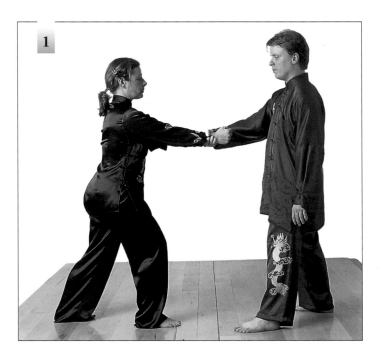

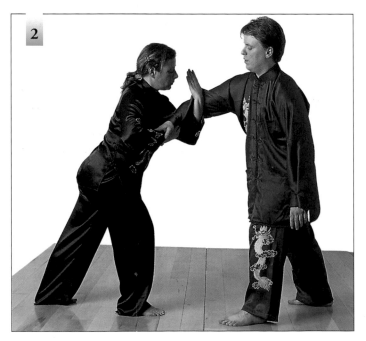

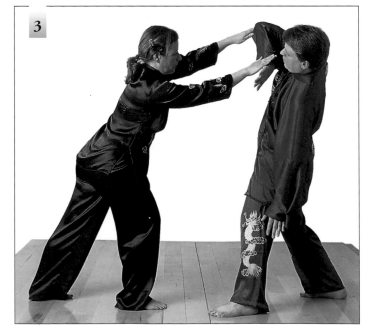

(25) CLOSING FORM

The Closing Form will bring us back into the original state–Wu Chi. After your expansion into the moves of the sequence, you return to the original void. The difference this time is that you have gained something inside yourself that is called Spirit.

THE MOVEMENT

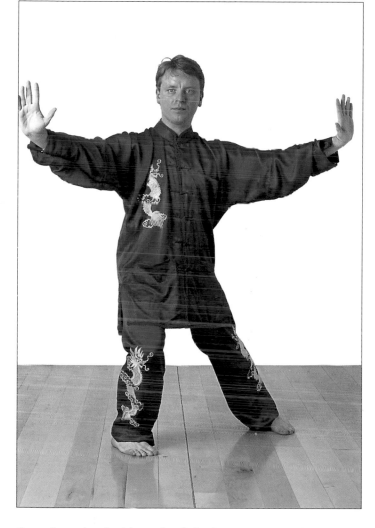

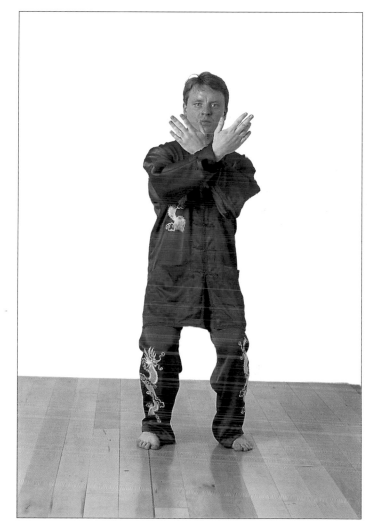

Start from the double push of the last movement. Move your waist in a clockwise direction and open your toes to the right. This will move your body weight onto your right leg. As your body weight moves, open your arms.

Turn your left toes so that they point in the direction that you are facing. Step back with your right leg so that you are in the parallel stance. Cross your forearms in front of your chest.

full sequence of the
25 Movements

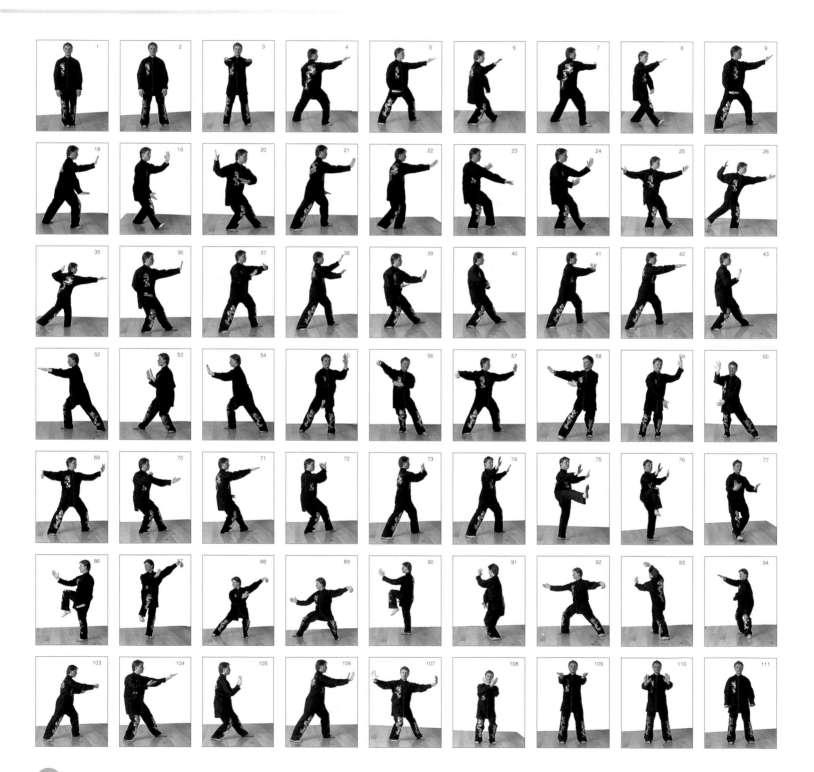

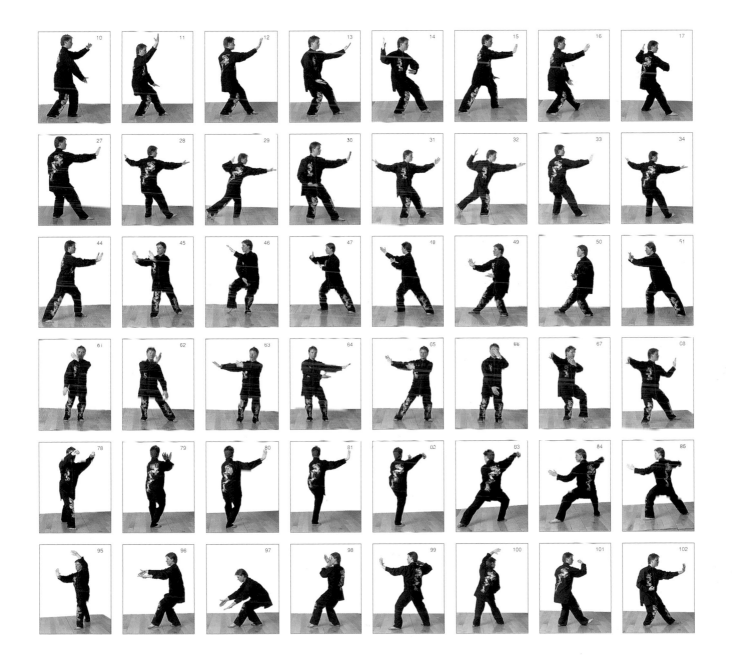

Conclusion

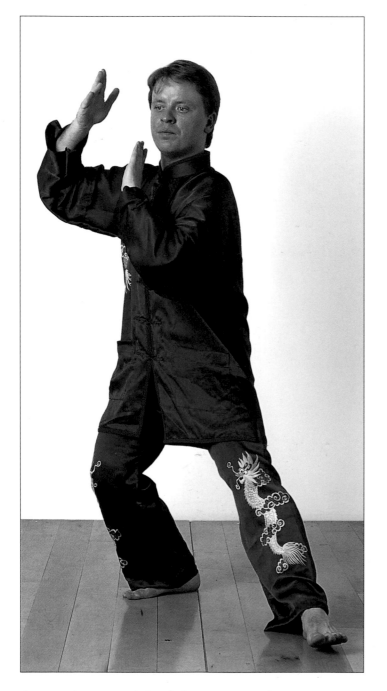

Practicing the moves regularly is the best way to master them

PRACTISING

When you have reached the end of the form, what next? Before you move on towards other aspects of Tai Chi, it is better to increase your skill with what you already know. Learning the sequence is relatively easy when compared to performing it correctly.

The Tai Chi Master, Chen Man Ching, stated that, as he saw it, there are three important factors that one needs to become skilled in Tai Chi. These are:

(1) Practice
(2) A good teacher
(3) Natural ability

Practice is the most important of the three factors. Natural ability is the least important on the list. We all have the ability to achieve good levels of success with Tai Chi, provided that we are prepared to do the practice. The only real natural ability is the ability to fit some practice into your daily routine.

The majority of modern people have tight daily schedules. If you find that you are enjoying Tai Chi, and want to make some real progress, you need to learn efficient ways of practising. If you simply do not have the time for long practice sessions, it is important to make the ones that you do get count.

The first thing to do is to set reasonable goals. Take small, but manageable steps. After one practice session for your Tai Chi, your skill level will not dramatically change. It is better to practice for a short time, but often, than to have long sessions infrequently.

Try to find time in your day to practice, even if it is only for a quarter of an hour. This will save you from having to repeat the same adjustments and improvements time and time again.

A successful approach is to pick out a movement and practice that particular move. You can pick any part of the form that you like for this approach. Now practice that movement until you really know it. You will find that there are many layers of knowledge for each movement.

When you pick on a movement in this way, it will influence the whole of your Tai Chi form. You will understand the feelings behind that movement and apply them to the rest of your form without even thinking about it. This process is sometimes called parallel learning. Working on one part in-depth will affect all of your other moves in parallel. The alternative would be to work more superficially on one move after the other in a more serial approach. The serial approach is usually slower and gives less insight into the deeper aspects of Tai Chi.

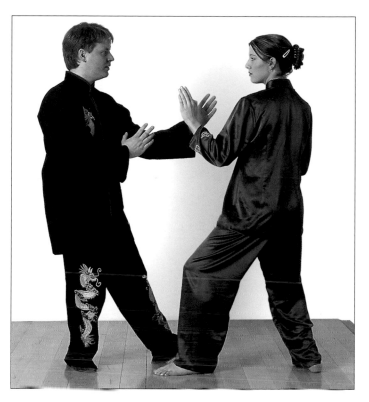

You will soon learn how effective 'softness' is against 'force'.

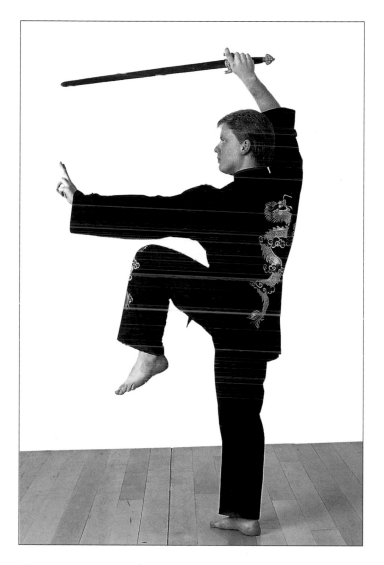

Weapons practice is a good next step if you wish to take your Tai Chi training further.

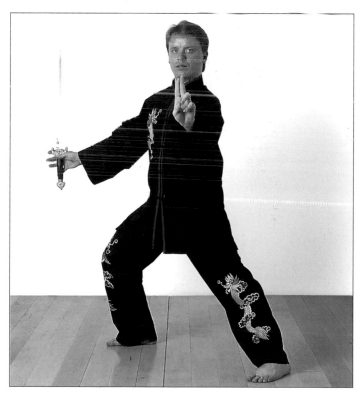

Learning to use a sword in Tai Chi will enhance your balance and co-ordination.

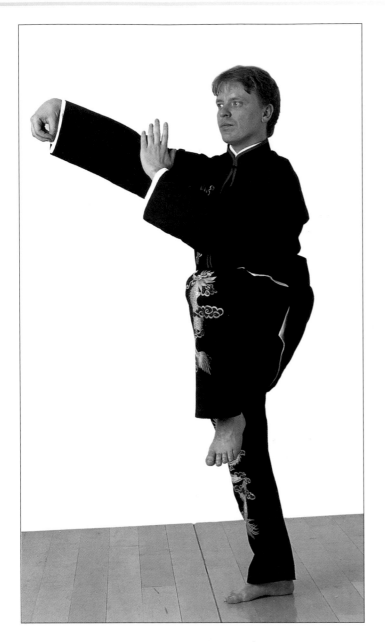

Regular practice will deepen you understanding of Tai Chi, allowing you to 'Lift Your Spirit'

DEVELOPMENTS

You have spent some time working on the moments, so what comes next? Tai Chi encompasses many fields of knowledge. When you have a good feeling for the basics, you may wish to explore further.

A logical progression after learning the simplified form is to learn the traditional Yang style form. This form contains one hundred and three separate movements. There are, however, many repetitions of the same movements. The transitions between the moves are where work will be required. In the Simplified Form that we have learned, there are twenty-four different movements. In the traditional Yang style Form there are eleven movements that will not have done before. Even with these new movements, the same basic Energies apply. It should be obvious that a good grounding in the Simplified Form will be priceless if you ever learn the traditional Yang form.

Other developments could include weapons training. Weapons training, such as learning to use a Tai Chi sword, forces you to be very accurate with your movements. If you are slightly out of alignment with your body, the alignment is magnified when you hold a weapon.

The lessons of Tai Chi become worthwhile when you can apply them to your daily life. The advantages of good posture are well documented and generally fairly obvious. A less obvious advantage is the idea of not using force. Aggressive situations can appear frequently, especially if you are surrounded by stress-sufferers in your workplace. As a change from becoming involved with their argument cycles you may wish to use a Tai Chi approach, and let them get on with it themselves. This can save you from being drawn into their arguments, and you will be more efficient through your day and less exhausted when you get home.

BLAZING TRUMPET, GRAND FINALE FINISH

If Tai Chi can help you regain inner balance, it is contagious. If you have ever met a high level Tai Chi Master, you will know that they seem to exude some sort of calmness around them. If you have not met anybody like this, think about the other extreme. If you know somebody who is frequently angry, you will have seen how he or she seems to bring the anger out in other people.

So you can see that on a metaphysical level, we are affecting the Energy of the whole Universe when we practice Tai Chi. This all boils down to the most important lesson that Tai Chi or any other discipline can teach us—LIFT THE SPIRIT!

Index

Picture credits:
ACE Photo Agency: pp 7t, 10, 23b
ET Archive: p9
Sarah Harris: p12b

All other pictures © Quantum Books Ltd

Many thanks to the models:
Anita, Maria, Paula, Rob.

The publisher and author would also like
to thank Le Huynh for supplying the
Tai Chi outfits used in the photographs.